teach your baby

the joys of water –

from newborn

floating

to toddler

swimming

water Babies

françoise barbira freedman

photography by christine hanscomb

forewords by david bance and virginia hunt newman

SELECT
EDITIONS

To Dadou, my star water baby

Select Editions imprint specially
produced for Selectabook Limited

© Anness Publishing Limited 2001
Updated © 2002

Produced by Anness Publishing Limited
Hermes House
88–89 Blackfriars Road
London SE1 8HA

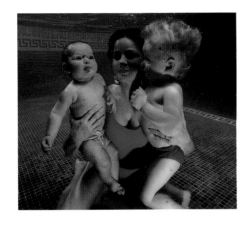

A CIP catalogue record for this book
is available from the British Library.

Publisher: Joanna Lorenz
Managing Editor: Helen Sudell
Project Editors: Melanie Halton, Debra Mayhew
Designer: Lisa Tai
Photographer: Christine Hanscomb
Editorial Reader: Richard McGinlay

10 9 8 7 6 5 4 3 2 1

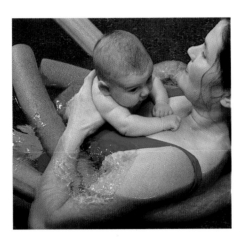

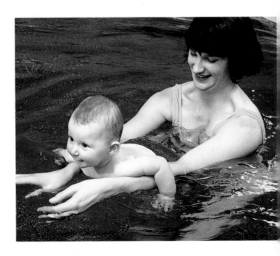

Contents

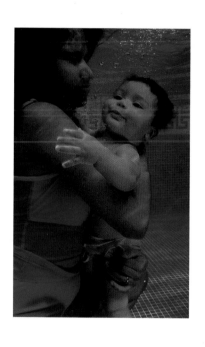

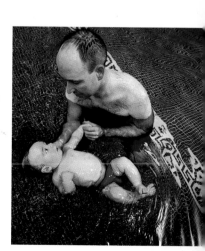

Forewords

TEACHING YOUR CHILD TO SWIM is one of life's true pleasures. It is an activity that plays a major part in the bonding process between the parent and the child. I'm sure we all remember the excitement and anticipation we felt as parents on first placing our child in water. Did they smile, cry or scream? Most mothers and fathers follow their parenting instincts, giving a cuddle, a kiss and lots of encouragement until the child gets used to entering the water. Many parents, however, just don't know what to do, and some transmit their fears and lack of confidence to their child.

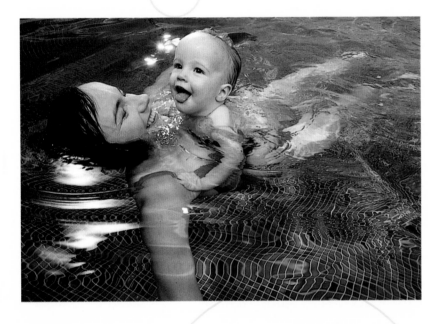

△ Teaching your baby the joys of swimming is a bonding and fun experience for both parent and child.

Your baby's introduction to water, from the very first bath to the first visit to a pool or a beach, should be one of fun and happiness. It is important to ensure that your child is confident and content in this new water environment, as these early experiences provide the foundation for the development of invaluable aquatic skills.

Fear not, help is at hand with Françoise Freedman's *Water Babies.* This well-illustrated, step-by-step guide presents very clear explanations of the essential early practices of aquatic development. I'm sure it will make a new and major contribution to the field of children's aquatic skills development, both for parents who wish to encourage their child to become comfortable in water and for the teaching professional. Indeed, *Water Babies* will assist the very foundation of aquatic sport from early development through to the elite athlete who has been taught the correct fundamental skills from an early age.

David Bance

Senior Coach for the British *Amateur Swimming Association*

THIS DELIGHTFUL BOOK is a guide to teaching babies from birth to three years of age to paddle through the water. It shows a loving, gentle approach to introducing babies to the the joys of buoyancy, helping them to develop a fondness for water that will last a lifetime.

During the 1930s, Myrtle McGraw PhD, at the University of Wisconsin, USA, compared the development of different species of animals, including a human baby, and demonstrated that each could "swim" through the water unassisted. A human baby, however, can only paddle a few feet because, at birth, his head is one-third the weight of his body so he is unable to raise it out of the water to breathe. This is one of the skills that he must be taught.

Between 1974 and 1977, Liselot Diem, then Federal Minister for Education and Science at the University of Cologne in Germany, taught swimming to babies. During this period, she investigated the effect of early motor stimulation on the total development of four to six-year-old children in comparison with a control group.

"Clearly evident and statistically born out, children who started to swim in their third month:

1. Showed an earlier and greater disposition for contacts, integrated faster and earlier into a peer group and were able to overcome disappointments caused by playmates more readily.

2. Were more independent and less fearful when confronted by new situations.

3. Showed better results in regard to intellectual ability and performance than the children in the comparison groups. Had greater precision in motion, better co-ordination and better balance."

Having taught infant swimming since the early 1950s, I can attest to the remarkable advantages and the wonderful contribution it can make to your child's personal development. As such, I believe that this informative book is a must for every parent who wishes to nurture a special bonding with their wee ones.

Virginia Hunt Newman

Founder of the *World Aquatic Babies Congress*

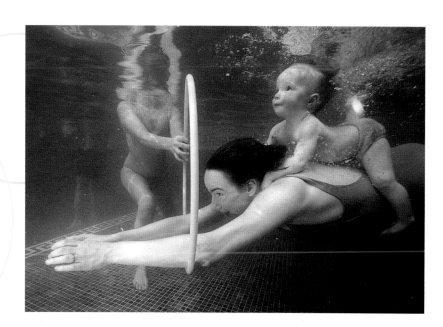

▷ **Early swimming skills will help your baby to develop strength, co-ordination and confidence.**

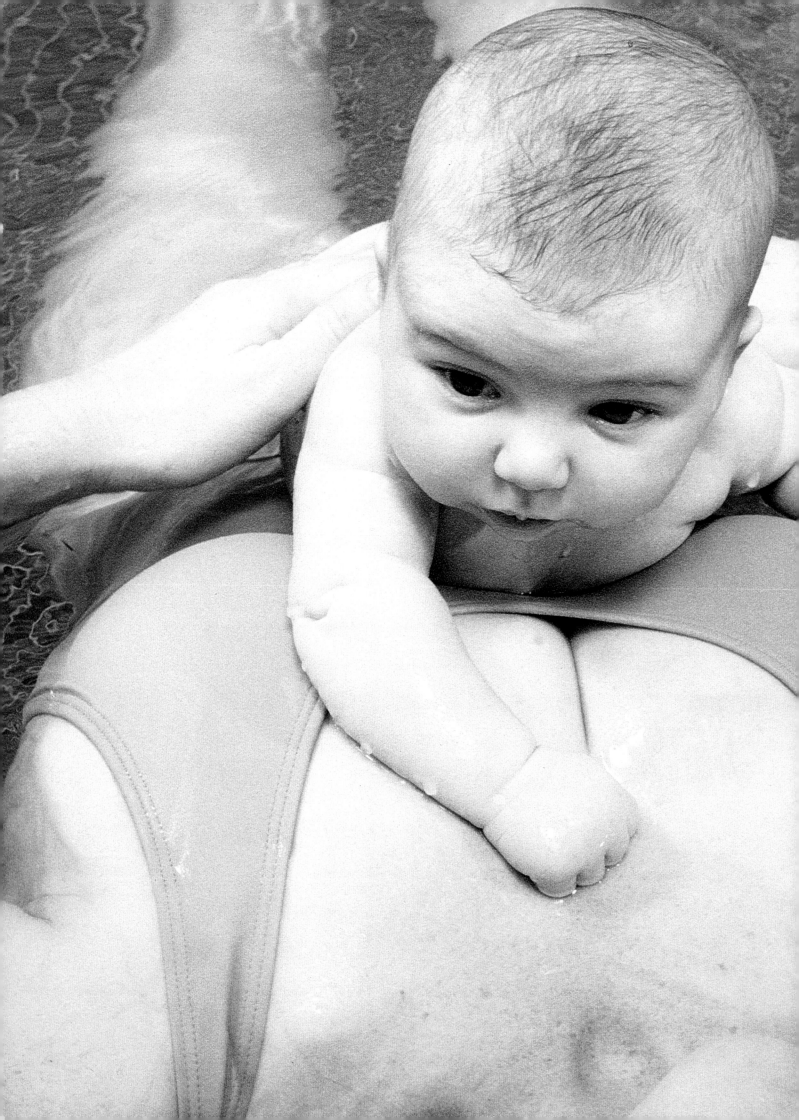

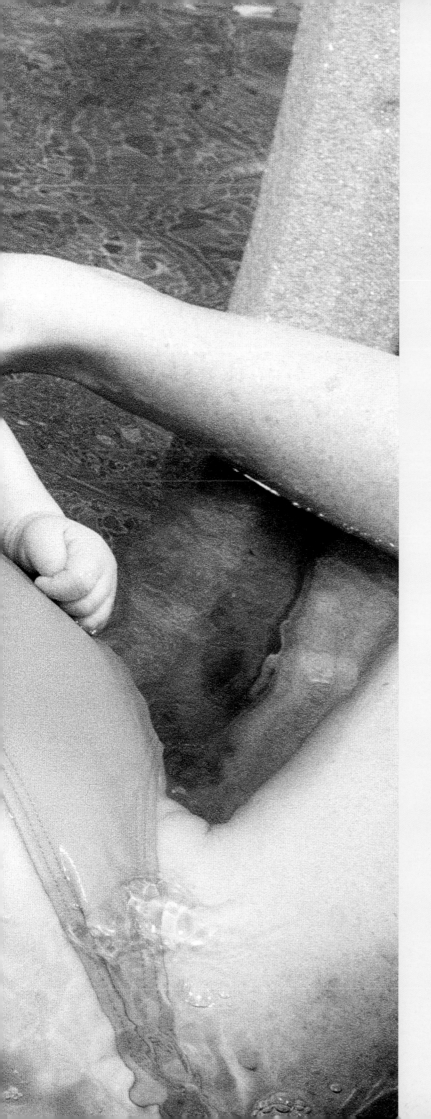

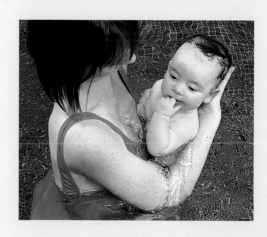

introducing
water
babies

Newborn babies are naturally at home in water, having spent nine months in the amniotic fluid of the womb. Playing together in water is an excellent way for parents to relax and begin bonding with their new child. It also helps to develop the child's physical and mental skills as well as their self-confidence.

A few opening words

My inspiration for *Water Babies* comes from the Upper Amazon. In the 1970s, I spent many happy afternoons in the river pools with forest people and their children at the daily bathtime, and it was a delight to watch parents train their babies to swim in a light-hearted and playful manner. I later became aware of the pioneers of infant swimming around the world. Their methods, combined with careful experimentation with my own four children, enabled me to develop the *Birthlight* approach described in this book. My main goal is to pass on to Western parents the happy attitude to babies in water that people, such as Amazonians and Polynesians, who live near warm water, are lucky enough to possess. Developing water confidence makes floating and swimming with babies bliss for them and for you.

how to use this book

This book presents integrated sets of exercises to do with your baby in water. In different and complementary ways, they strengthen your baby and consolidate early swimming reflexes into swimming movements. Successive exercises in each set suit different age groups from birth,

EACH SESSION SHOULD INCLUDE AND COMBINE THE FOUR FOLLOWING ACTIVITIES:

• Holding your baby in the water in positions that stimulate movement of the legs and later the arms.
• Swimming with your baby, so that he experiences and registers the motions of swimming close to your body.
• Going underwater, by submerging, diving or jumping.
• Playing games related to skills as well as for fun.

A relatively fast pace works best for most babies so that they are never bored.

developing skills in gradually more expanded versions. According to the age of your baby when you take her to the pool, choose the level of practice and move on from there, taking your time to complete each stage. You need to give more attention to the security of an older baby, particularly for submersion, in order to consolidate happy experiences.

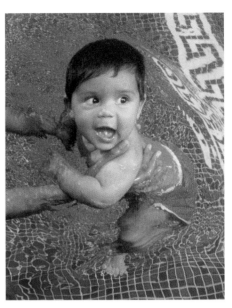

△ **Feeling happy and secure in the water is the foundation of swimming.**

Each section starts with gentle movements suitable for either very young babies or older babies who have just been introduced to water. At first, try one or two of these exercises. As you and your baby get more confident, progress through the more advanced versions. Combine the exercises to compose your own session.

A session in warm water should last 10 to 20 minutes for a baby under 12 weeks and 30 to 35 minutes for older babies. Start with holding and floating, then swimming, submersion and play at the level that suits your baby. While young babies are happy with the same activity for up to 10 minutes, babies over 6 months need a greater range. Do not stand idle with babies of any age in the water (for example, talking to another parent) – always float or move in the water. If you want to take a small break, it is better to go to the steps and sit to cuddle your baby or play with him on the edge or in the water.

You can use this book either in parent and baby swimming sessions or on your own or with friends. Inform the instructor,

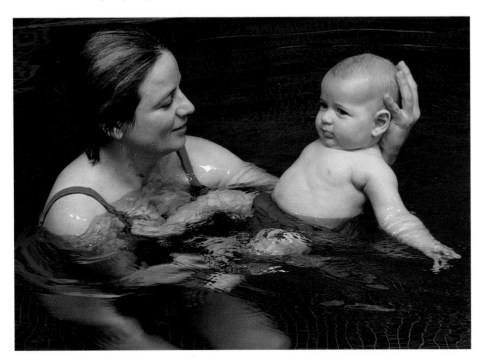

◁ **Water enables parents to communicate with their babies without any distractions.**

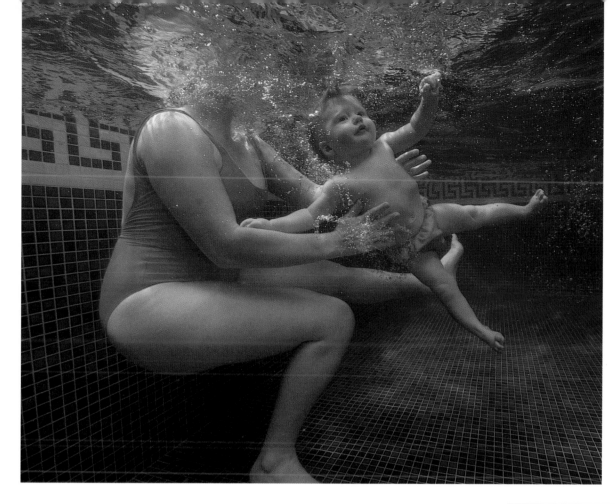

◁ **Early submersions help your baby to be totally at ease in the water. Most toddlers start swimming underwater and surface to breathe.**

group leader or pool supervisor that you wish to practise exercises with your baby that include submersion, and make sure that he or she agrees beforehand (pools have specific policies concerning what is allowed in parent and baby classes).

how often to go

No baby has a smooth, even progression towards unaided swimming. This is why it is important for success that you take your baby to the pool regularly, at least once a week but preferably twice. Daily swims during vacations often result in a leap forward in babies' progress. Your commitment as a "water parent" will be put to the test by the plateaus on which your baby or toddler will seem to be stuck for what seems an eternity, until the next breakthrough finally occurs beyond your expectations. Expect a regression between weeks three and four when you introduce a baby over four months to the pool, sometimes with quite a strong reaction. Do not get discouraged and think that your baby does not like water, since this seems to be part of a common adjustment process. If your baby is still unhappy at the pool after week four but happy generally, ask your doctor to check your baby's ears and skin. If

your baby enjoys the bath but not the pool, try changing pools and start again from the first gentle introductory movements.

Regularity is most important for babies. If you miss up to four weeks' swimming with a baby under six months, start again from earlier gentle movements, particularly if your baby has been unwell. If you miss more than a month with a baby below the age of one, the transition from reflex movements to conscious movements may have been interrupted and you may have to make greater use of supporting floats than you would have otherwise. Routines also matter; babies remember the pool vividly from an early age and build up associations from week to week. Activities that babies and toddlers perceive to be part of swimming, such as socializing in the changing room and a snack afterwards, increase their pleasure and anticipation.

The main focus of this book is to allow your baby to discover buoyancy through feeling and understanding the water. At every stage in your baby's development, your challenge is to offer as little support as possible in the water until your baby shows signs of being ready to take off. All along, respect your baby's unique pace, and lavish praise, love and trust.

SOME BASIC RECOMMENDATIONS

• Avoid giving your baby mixed messages, particularly if you have an intrinsic fear of water. Make a statement that you are getting used to this, or you are being very brave here, rather than trying to hide your feelings. Your panic will add to your baby's possible fear. Every time you experience this fear again, acknowledging it will help you gradually overcome it.

• Set clear rules at the pool about what is permissible and what is not. Take action firmly, without alarm, when babies start hoisting themselves from the pool, tottering on the steps or standing precariously on the edge. Interrupting the dangerous new game and moving on immediately to another activity works better than loud "no"s for conveying that pools have a particular set of rules that must be followed.

• Always leave on a happy note. Just as with beginnings, endings are important to create happy memories. Babies like saying goodbye to the pool.

The benefits of *early* swimming

The benefits of early swimming are manifold, and helping babies along the way to swimming can be one of parents' most enjoyable experiences. Infants make an easy transition from their early swimming reflexes to conscious movement if you swim with them and show them how to find their buoyancy in the water with minimal support. The emphasis is on encouraging free movement in water that is conducive to swimming at such a time when your baby is both physically and emotionally ready.

However, it is not just a case of playing in the water with your baby; there is a carefully designed progression of skills based on many years of experience with a wide range of babies in the water in *Birthlight* classes.

motivation

Perhaps you are an avid swimmer and you wish to teach your baby to swim as early as possible. Maybe you were frightened as a child while learning to swim, but you wish your baby to feel good in water, and perhaps overcome your own fear in the process. Perhaps, after having a waterbirth, you feel that your baby may have an innate affinity for water. It could simply be that water as an element attracts you, and you see it as a medium in which you can play with your baby actively and promote sound development, health and good fun. If you follow the various sequences presented in the book, your baby will start swimming as a

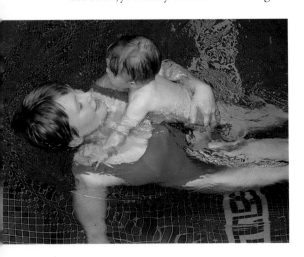

matter of course. This occurs exceptionally at the end of the first year but more frequently in the second year and sometimes in the third year. Basic water safety skills are acquired along the way, matching your baby's development.

parental closeness and involvement

The interaction of parents with babies in the water underlies all the short-term and long-term benefits of early swimming. The focus is on mutual enjoyment: the more that babies take pleasure in early swimming, the more delighted are their parents and the more the babies thrive.

a gentle approach

A baby who is not immediately happy in water can be gently coaxed with loving, focused encouragement and without pressure. The main benefit of such a gentle approach is to give babies a model about acquiring major skills in a playful mode without trauma. This may remain imprinted in their psyche for use later on in life. It is more effective to show by example or repeatedly remove babies from what is dangerous or unwanted, rather than coerce or reinforce responses through commands.

◁ **Babies who need security can continue taking rides until they feel ready to let go.**

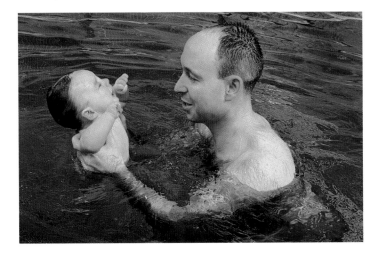

◁ **In water, fathers can get to know their babies in a playful and relaxed mode. Swimming can be the first sport you have fun with together and can be enjoyed for a lifetime.**

This is more feasible in water, where babies have our undivided attention, than in the hurly burly of daily life on dry land.

the mutual benefit

You, the parent, also benefit from your baby's early swimming in many ways. Forget about "teaching" your baby to swim: if you have a loving, happy time with your baby in the water, enjoying the water, the second goal will take care of itself. The trick is not to separate them: having fun and swimming go together. Going swimming together helps you to get to know your baby better and may help consolidate bonding, whether you are the mother or the father. It may help you come to terms with an intrinsic fear of water. It may help you recover a playfulness you have not experienced since childhood. It may teach you how to adapt to your baby's personality for best results.

physiological benefits

There is no conclusive research, but professionals involved in waterbirth or in "baby swimming" programmes claim that babies exposed to water early are happier and healthier than other babies. German researchers have shown that early swimmers perform better on tests measuring social, academic, motor and personality developments, although such

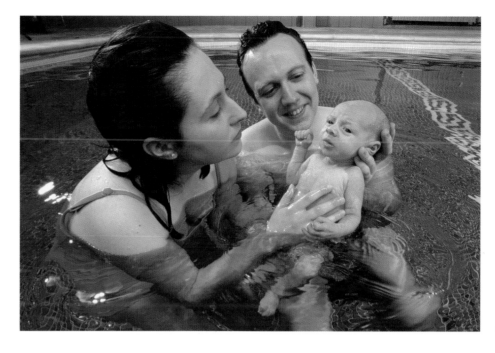

results may also be attributed to the overall quality of parenting. Babies who develop their swimming abilities are often more alert for their age, with a better eating and sleeping pattern. In addition, just as for adults, swimming improves babies' cardio-respiratory function and general health.

Russian researchers claim that the energy used on land to fight the force of gravity can be freed in water after birth and used for three purposes: to develop the body and above all the brain, which is most receptive and active in the period following birth; to investigate the environment and acquire different kinds of knowledge as babies move freely in three dimensions; and to create new brain functions, which facilitate problem solving and task handling.

Babies can exercise more muscles in the weightless water environment, as they are not restricted by their incapacity to sit or stand up. This earlier strength manifests itself in an early ability to raise themselves up using their arms and in walking.

The transformation of reflex movement into conscious movement in the water may facilitate early co-ordination. Babies develop balance as they learn to roll and move bilaterally in water to maintain their equilibrium, crucial for later swimming.

In addition, water offers babies a heightened multi-sensory stimulation involving touch, hearing, sight, taste and smell. The intense physical contact and eye contact with parents also offer quality stimulation. This can be especially valuable for premature or special-needs babies.

psychological development

Early swimming helps to develop babies' personalities harmoniously; cautious babies learn to accept risk while rumbustious babies learn to be more prudent. As babies discover that they can propel themselves in the water, their independence and self-confidence increase. Water offers them opportunities to respond to the unexpected early on. Toddlers are delighted with their achievements and readily show their enjoyment to parents and others in the pool.

safety

Drowning is the second greatest cause of accidental death in children in industrialized countries. More than 50 per cent of cases of drowning occur close to the water's edge. No method of infant swimming can guarantee to safeguard against drowning, but your baby has a better chance of survival if familiarity with water allows her to remain relaxed in case of an accidental fall.

Once a baby can swim back to the edge after jumping into the pool, in principle she has become water-safe, but it will take a few more months to consolidate her safety skills. You need to remain watchful. Swimming toddlers are often at risk from becoming over-confident. During the transition period when infants start to swim unaided but cannot yet surface to breathe, extra caution is needed at all times.

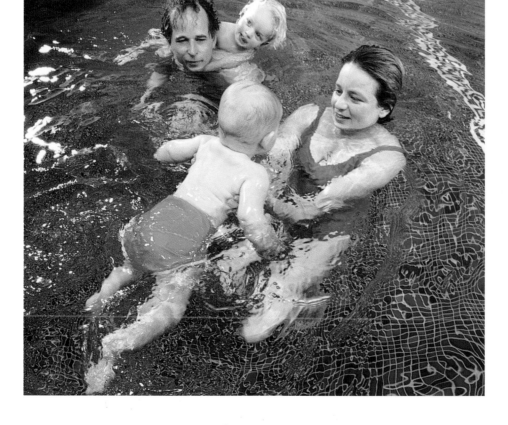

Frequently asked questions

To be relaxed with your baby and have a happy experience, you need to be informed. Parents who start swimming with their babies tend to ask the same questions, which mostly refer to safety, conditions and performance.

is it safe for babies to go underwater?

This book supports the belief that babies hold their breath when submerged in their first half year, that their bodies are designed to conserve oxygen automatically, and that when newborns are exposed to water, they make automatic swimming movements. (However, there are opponents of baby swimming who claim that, after birth, being in water ceases to be a natural function.)

Two main responses are triggered when your baby goes underwater. Firstly, the diving response: whenever babies' faces are in the water, the circulating blood starts to conserve oxygen and utilize it most efficiently. Oxygenated blood is directed to sustain the brain and heart for as long as 30 minutes. Not only submersion but simple immersions of the baby's face elicit this "diving response". Babies that are submersed for only seconds at a time a few times per session are not exposed to any risk. Secondly, there is the "gag reflex" (laryngospasm). When water gets into your baby's mouth, the gag reflex causes an involuntary spasm of the glottis and the epiglottis, keeping water from entering the trachea (windpipe). This watertight seal of the windpipe prevents inhalation of water into the lungs.

Remember, however, that the gag reflex does not close off the esophagus and water can accumulate in your baby's stomach, with the possibility of causing water intoxication. Parents must watch that their infants do not swallow a lot of water when they are held prone. The risk of intoxication is, however, extremely remote in a half-hour session in which you practise a variety of exercises, even if your baby tends to swallow water. Water intoxication is a rare condition. Unlike near drowning, no water has entered the lungs. Symptoms are lethargy, irritability and nausea. Consult your doctor if you are concerned.

when can babies start?

From birth to nine months, babies adjust easily to a water environment. The later babies are introduced to the water, the more likely they are to object to the unfamiliar sensations and thus experience fear. In my experience, the best time to start is between six and 16 weeks. Many parents like to wait until their babies have had their immunizations and are considered to be protected from polio, but consult your doctor for advice if needed.

Although it is best to introduce your baby to water as early as possible, you should

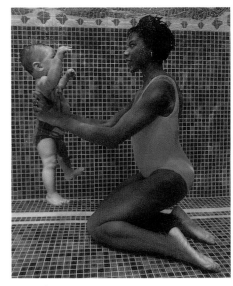

△ **Most babies are happy to go underwater, particularly if you are in sight.**

never feel under pressure to go to a pool. It is in fact possible for you and your baby to achieve a great deal at home in the bath.

LARYNGEAL REFLEX (GAG REFLEX) AND DIVING RESPONSE

The introduction of water in the upper airway of newborns and infants arrests respiration through triggering a complex reflex at the entrance to the larynx. An involuntary spasm causes the epiglottis to close over the larynx, creating a watertight seal and preventing inhalation of water into the lungs via the trachea. There are many similarities between the cardiovascular adjustments in this early reflex and in the diving response, which is stimulated when babies' faces are immersed in the water. Both serve to protect life by directing declining oxygenated blood to the brain and heart when breathing is interrupted.

Please note:

• The gag reflex prevents babies from inhaling water but it does not close off the esophagus, which leads to the stomach. Babies occasionally swallow water, some more than others. Long and frequent submersions, which can cause water intoxication, are therefore not advisable.

• Some babies have a stronger diving response than others and this response also diminishes with age. Between nine and 36 months there is a delicate transition to breath-holding which then triggers cardiovascular adjustments during diving.

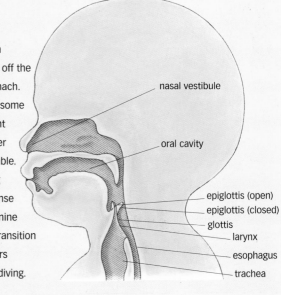

nasal vestibule

oral cavity

epiglottis (open)
epiglottis (closed)
glottis
larynx
esophagus
trachea

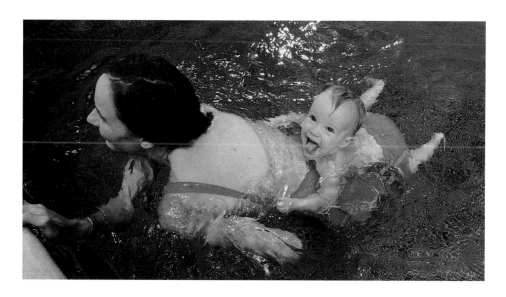

◁ There can be a long period when your baby seems ready to swim and yet does not want to take off. Ultimately, it's your baby's decision. Each baby's progression is unique.

when will my baby swim?

Many parents expect their babies to be able to swim soon after they are introduced to the water. It all depends on what is meant by swimming. While some infants may move freely in water after just a few sessions, it is very rare that they become able to swim unaided to a target before entering their second year. By focusing on enjoying being in water with your baby as your main goal, you avoid putting pressure on achievement and expecting quick results, both of which are often counter-productive.

Some parents are under the impression that their babies will float from birth; very few babies do, if any. Helping your baby to develop full buoyancy as he grows is part of the joy of swimming.

what if my baby does not like the water?

Each baby is different. Some newborns like water more than others, usually those with a higher proportion of fatty tissue. Mind your reactions and your words if your baby cries in the bath or the pool. Rather than jump to the conclusion that he does not like water, check that the temperature is warm enough, comfort him and aim to create pleasurable associations each time you expose him to water again.

is a baby's health at risk in the water?

Well-maintained, monitored and cared-for public pools pose fewer threats to your baby's health than your bath tub or private pools. Bacteria that thrive in hot water are a low hazard because of chlorine's effectiveness in pools. Take more precautions with young babies in lakes and on beaches – because of

environmental pollution – and babies who have not been immunized against polio are more at risk.

Babies who swim are not more likely to have ear infections. Unless your baby has a perforated eardrum, it is not possible for water in the outer canal to flow into the middle or inner ear where ear infections start. Simple preventive habits with your baby after swimming are very helpful; after getting out of the pool, turn your baby to each side to drain any water from his ears before drying them well with a towel. Put a woollen hat on your baby before going outdoors in cold or wet, windy weather.

Unless your baby has a sniffly cold, a chest infection, an ear or an eye infection, going swimming is unlikely to worsen any mild condition. In fact, swimming can clear common colds and be invigorating, and it is recommended medically as the best exercise for asthmatic children since it does not produce bronchial hyperactivity.

Babies who have eczema may not be able to swim in chlorinated pools. After a couple of trials, you will know whether your baby's condition is made worse by swimming, and you may wish to take medical advice.

how much time should I leave between feeding and swimming?

Young babies can be fed at any time, including immediately before getting into the water. They rarely regurgitate milk or vomit in the water. Older babies who are fed solid food, however, may bring it up in the

▷ You can feed your baby at the side of the pool, immediately before entering the water.

water if they have eaten just before swimming, particularly if they have mucus in their stomachs. If your baby tends to do this, avoid snacks before going to the pool but make sure you take a healthy snack with you for after swimming.

Loud burps in the water are to be expected from babies. Cheer your baby! If he gets hiccups, avoid submersion, as it may cause him to swallow water.

what if my baby soils the pool?

Do not let this possibility worry you excessively. You can expect it to occur once, perhaps twice, in your baby's first two years of regular swimming. If it happens, stay calm, remove your baby from the pool without communicating alarm or worry. Small amounts of faecal matter will be quickly filtered or netted out of the water. Some pools change the water after an "incident", while others do not. Whatever the policy, remember that it can happen to anyone and make sure that you see the funny side of it. Baby swimming diapers are now available in many stores and are practical.

can parents who cannot swim teach their babies to swim?

Many parents who are not confident in water are motivated to help their babies swim without fear. It is a positive step. Make sure, however, that you can be relaxed enough so as to regain your footing easily in case you slip while holding your baby.

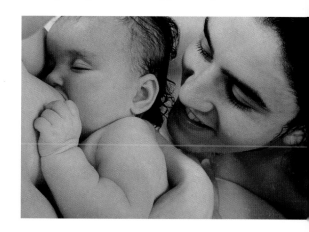

Natural swimming reflexes

Recent photographs of young babies underwater and looking relaxed with no adult in sight give the impression that the babies are swimming or totally amphibian. This is misleading, because babies need to gain strength and control to raise themselves to the surface in order to breathe. Babies under eight months cannot do this unaided. From birth to six months, they are primed to hold their breath and move their arms and legs in a reflexive way but they cannot use extended arms, leg kicks or lift their heads to breathe. If photographs of this kind have inspired you initially, you can now follow your baby through the process that will lead her from appearing to swim to actually swimming.

the *Birthlight* approach

This technique seeks to consolidate the baby's swimming reflexes and help them become conscious movements of legs and arms in water at the end of the first year. Most infant reflexes are outgrown after six months, unless they are sustained by regular active stimulation. The first step is to recognize your baby's reflexes. Then different positions are used to stimulate them,

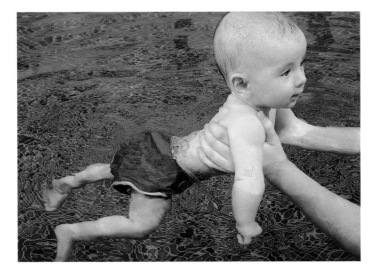

strengthen them and help your baby produce them as movements. The more relaxed you are and the earlier you start, the stronger your baby's swimming reflexes are likely to be.

The *Birthlight* approach makes full use not only of babies' reflexive movements but also of their natural tendency to learn by imitation from the time they are born. Although it will take a year or so for your baby to imitate particular movements directly, month by month they will register what you do in the water and produce a gradually more refined imitation. This is

why it is easier to swim with babies than to "teach" them how to swim, to go underwater with them rather than merely to submerge them so that they hold their breath. If you cannot swim, the best course of action is to be open to discovering the water in a new way with your baby and acknowledge your fear until you are able to relax totally in the water.

the amphibian reflex

This is the newborn's most basic reflex in the water. It causes the legs, arms and torso to move in spurs that can propel the newborn through the water for a very short distance unaided. Reinforcing this reflex with practice in the pool between four and eight months helps your baby to make the transition from involuntary movement to voluntary leg kicking. It manifests both when babies are on their backs and when they are placed prone in the water with their face submerged, when they hold their breath automatically. Babies who follow the practices in this book will start generating their own movement in the water and so will not sink, motionless, when the reflex phases out between five and seven months.

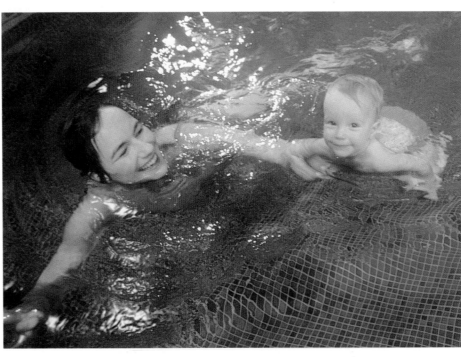

⊲ As your baby starts swimming beside you, supported by your arm or a woggle (swim noodle), her movements become more co-ordinated.

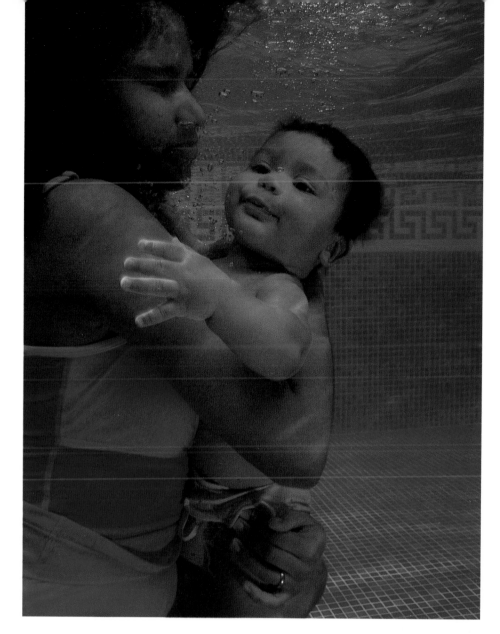

▷ Breath-holding is consolidated by regular practice during the first year. Babies learn to close their mouths in anticipation as they prepare to go underwater.

righting reflex

When an infant over four or five months is lying on her back in the water, she will try to bring her head back to an upright position. Babies lying on their front will also tend to keep their heads upright above the water. These movements of the head are part of the "righting reflex". Floating exercises aim at avoiding the stimulation of this reflex by supporting the head of the baby and ensure that she will continue to enjoy swimming on her back, as well as floating, through her second year. Most babies learn to swim on their front and tend to roll from their backs to a prone position. A few babies first learn swimming on their backs, and occasionally a baby will start swimming in either position.

reflexive holding of the breath

The diving response and gag reflex gradually give way to learned association through practice from the start. If it is practised regularly, learned breath-holding is consolidated during the first year and remains an acquired skill for life. Long interruptions in the course of the first year may, however, compromise this learning.

follow your baby's development in the water

This book is ideally suited for babies under one year old, although it can be used with older children, up to two years. The approach then has to be modified, however, because reflexes have been lost and fear of water may have been acquired. Relaxed holding, which is the main way of making young babies feel secure in the water, must be reinforced by verbal encouragement with older babies to allow them to adjust to the pool as an unfamiliar environment. A variety of exercises performed by parent and baby together initiate babies to swimming in a progressively more independent way as they grow stronger and more proficient. No baby's progress, however early the start, is ever totally smooth. There may be times when your baby seems to regress and clings to you, refusing to hold on to anything but your body in the water. This may last for weeks, sometimes months. You may come to think that your efforts to encourage your baby to swim early have been in vain, and you may be tempted to be discouraged, disenchanted and even give up altogether. It is precisely at this time, usually at the end of the first year and the beginning of the second, that it is most important to continue taking your baby to the pool even though there is no sign of progress. Babies who do not "take off" at the same time as they are learning to walk often need to consolidate their security in the water for what may seem a very long time, on their own terms, before deciding to swim. On that day, they may surprise you with a nearly perfect stroke!

Besides the known times when your baby is more likely to be affected by separation anxiety (around 7–9 months, 14–15 months), a mother's new pregnancy, a long journey, changes in baby care or tensions in the home may temporarily affect your baby's swimming. Learning to crawl, walk and talk may also change your baby's performance in the water in different ways, either speeding her progress or slowing it.

Whenever and in whichever way your baby makes the transition to swimming unaided, a close and happy interaction with parents in the water remains a priority through all stages of development. This is why in the *Birthlight* approach parents are encouraged to start with supported floating, because priority is given to relaxation in water with parents and experiencing movement in water with a relaxed attitude. Babies discover their ability to swim unaided because they continue to be relaxed enough to float and hold their breath underwater without anxiety. They then propel themselves in the water towards someone they know and love.

Water parenting

For millennia, populations living near warm water have encouraged their babies to start swimming by frolicking in shallow pools, perhaps washing clothes or vegetables at the same time. To Polynesian or Amazonian people, swimming is not a skill that has to be taught, but rather an ability, like walking, that is part of growing up. It can be stimulated and encouraged, but the learning is gradual and almost effortless. Remember that you are your baby's favourite meaningful person for some time to come. The mutual delight of moving in the water with you conveys to your baby at a deep level that you can be trusted and life is to be enjoyed. The patient, skilful and often lengthy apprenticeship that takes you and your baby along the way to unaided swimming is known as "water parenting". The early stages of water parenting can be the beginning of a lifelong process of sharing activities with your growing child.

quality time together

In the water, parents have the opportunity of uninterrupted, close time with their babies. Both fathers and mothers sometimes feel that being in water allows them to discover their babies in a new way. Infant swimming complements infant massage and baby yoga. While close physical contact is mediated by the water, responding with total attention makes your baby feel loved, self-confident, important, competent and gradually aware of his abilities and eager to exercise them in a self-motivated way.

If you were apprehensive about taking your baby swimming, you may now be more reassured by understanding how his reflexes operate. If your baby goes under for a few seconds he will possibly not mind at all unless you make a drama of it. When this happens, and it inevitably will, remember that the best thing you can do is to stay relaxed and gently bring your baby back to the surface without any panicky, sudden movements that may convey anxiety.

Enabling and encouraging your baby to swim while you too may be learning to relax in the water is a particular apprenticeship. Water intensifies the exchanges you have with your baby; it tests your responses and helps you to develop your parenting skills in unexpected ways. For this reason, creating a relaxed and stress-free atmosphere is a priority. Your baby will meet many of life's challenges in rapid succession in the water, and your response will help to shape his personality. With the *Birthlight* approach advocated in this book – that trust and love will get the best results – water parenting will be most enjoyable and probably most fruitful.

praising both successes and failures

Water parenting shows your baby that you love him unconditionally in practice, in a way that is not contingent on success and achievement. Skills are introduced gradually and never forced on crying babies. Praise, hugs, kisses and the joy of their accomplishments motivate babies to take on new challenges. Some babies resist certain activities, such as jumping or being submerged. While it is good to keep trying, introducing them at regular intervals as your baby grows and changes, do not feel that it is necessary to master any particular skill at a particular stage in order to swim unaided. It is when your baby shows resistance to an activity that you need to express your love for him the most. Not only is it generous, but it is an act of trust in your baby's future achievements. Often babies who are supported during phases when they seem to be "stuck" go on to overtake the babies who appeared most eager earlier on. Celebrating another baby's achievements when your baby appears to lag behind is also very positive. Respecting your baby's current attitude to water while keeping in mind that it may change completely in a matter of weeks or months can be difficult. Watching

▷ **Swimming with your baby promotes closeness and develops skills for later life.**

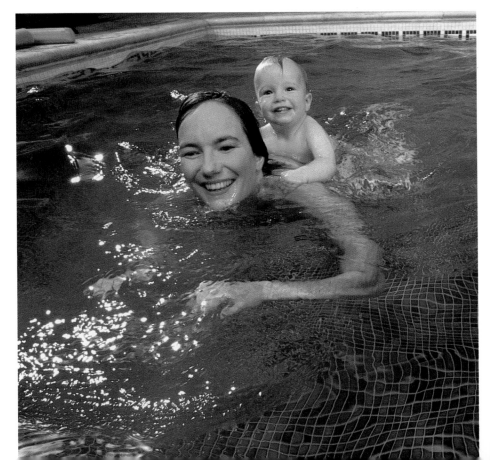

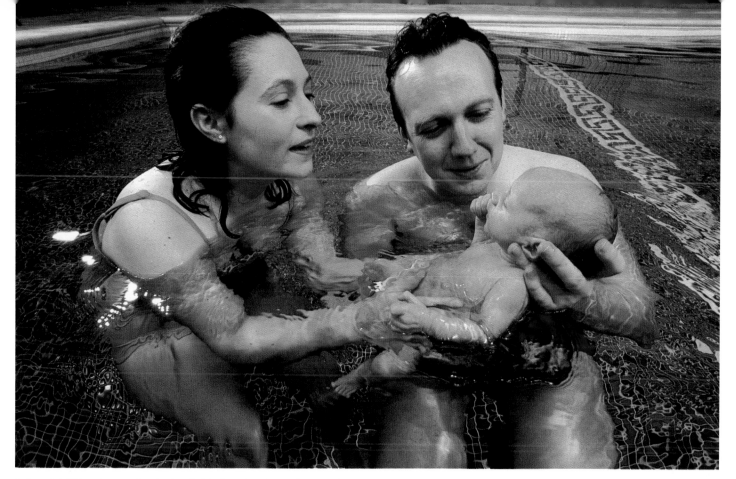

△ **Parents' different ways of caring for their infants in water can enrich the experience and create closer bonds within the whole family.**

your energetic and daring eight-month-old turn into a clinging limpet, even if you trust that it is temporary, may be a shock. Try not to become too disheartened, however, as your baby will progress at his own rate. Fears are short-lived if handled with understanding and encouragement rather than dismissed or repressed. Let your baby emerge afresh from each readjustment period, however long and trying it is, by offering incentives to overcome fear and praising each small breakthrough. In times of regression, it can be helpful to return to earlier gentle exercises and indulge your baby with what gives him the most pleasure in the water.

Keeping your sense of humour in the water is an essential parenting skill – it helps to eliminate unnecessary drama and creates a light-hearted atmosphere in the pool.

communication rather than commands

In the *Birthlight* approach, submersion is encouraged only to the extent that it is enjoyable for the baby. Rather than the commands on which drown-proofing (methods used to forcefully condition babies to survive alone in water while waiting for help) techniques rely and which

many swimming schools use to incite babies to hold their breath underwater, it is better to use signals that reinforce communication. Babies are encouraged to imitate parents non-verbally first, for example to hold their breath, before a verbal signal is added to create an association with this action. This is a subtle difference but one that has wide-ranging implications for the style of parenting to which your baby is getting accustomed. While some drown-proofed babies appear to have difficulties with co-ordinated swimming later on, babies who imitate parents and follow non-verbal cues early on also seem to be more receptive to improving their strokes through imitation as they grow older.

This way of teaching babies and young children is close to the way of aboriginal people around the world. It does not mean that you are not constantly encouraging the behaviour or skill you wish your baby to develop, but the motivation comes from the rewards rather than forceful habituation. If your baby cries, the response is always to stop and cuddle him before trying again what you were attempting. You

▷ **Watching, interpreting responses and signalling what comes next are all part of water parenting.**

should not think, however, that each time your baby cries, you cease encouraging a new skill. The difference is between pressure for achievement and low-key nudging and coaxing in a playful mode. Babies also need to discover gradually the consequences of their actions – for example that if they cease to hold on when swimming with you (over four months) they fall off into the water.

fathers and mothers

Water parenting requires a delicate balance between closeness and comfort on the one hand, and allowing your baby to be self-reliant and self-motivated on the other. Parents often have very different attitudes – one may be more protective, the other more daring. However, these different approaches can complement one another in the water.

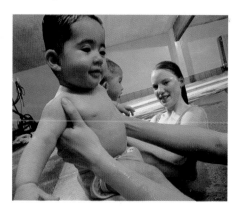

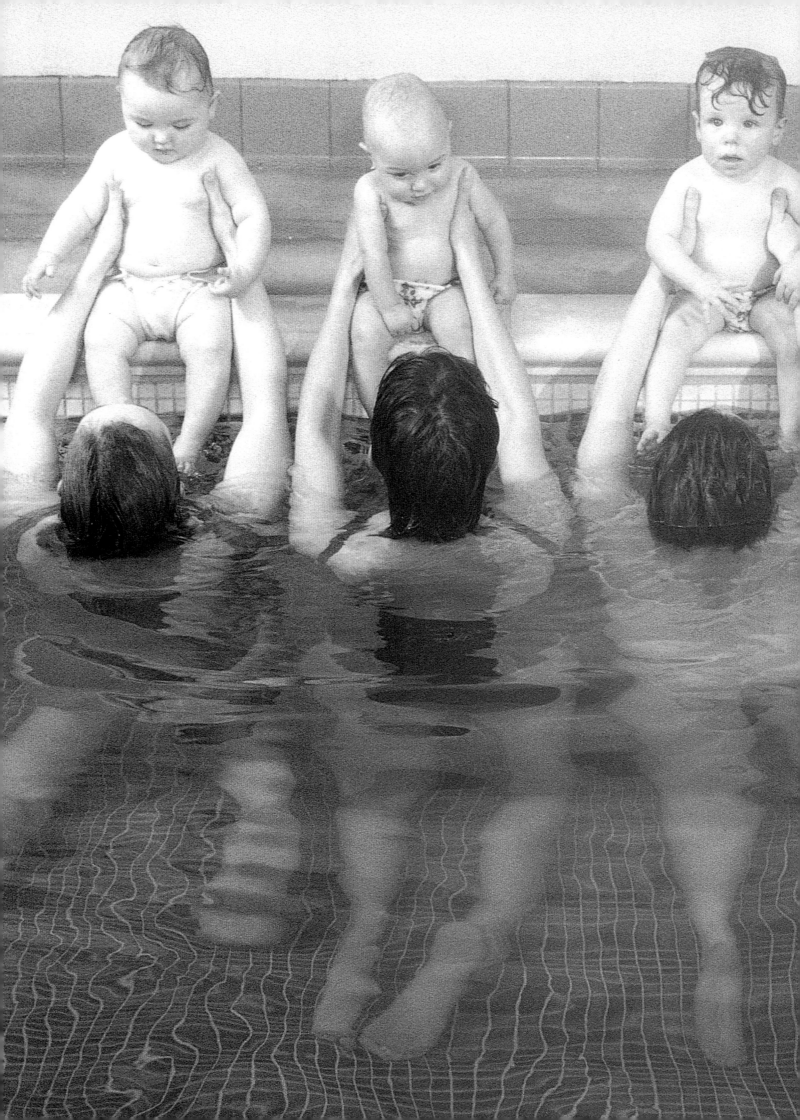

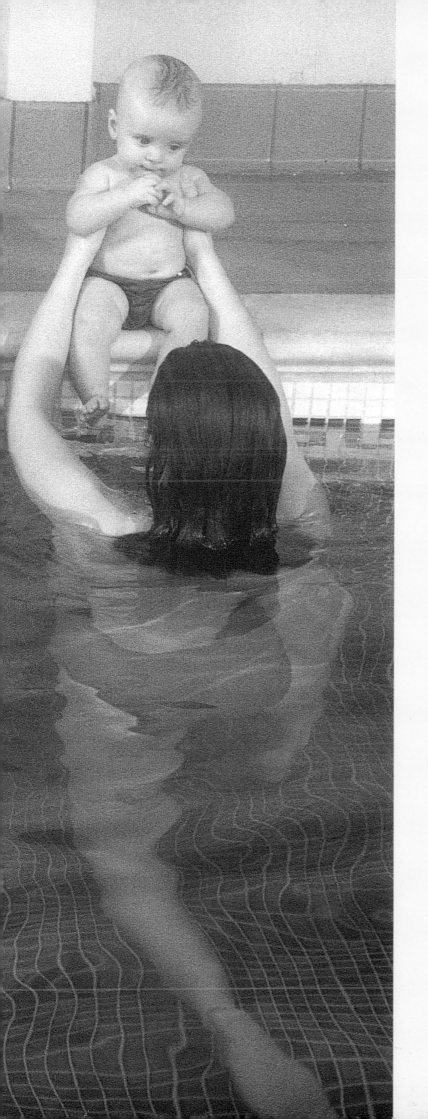

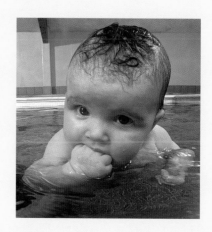

the early
stages

The parents of water babies do not have to be fast-lane swimmers or deep-sea divers. A happy, caring, yet carefree attitude conveys best to your baby that water is a different medium to play in – first at home in the bath and later on at the pool. Simple guidelines are required, not only for overall safety, but also to time and structure your sessions in a way that best suits your baby's age, temperament and mood.

Choosing a pool and equipment

No pool is perfect, but it is worth taking the time to look for a suitable pool near where you live, even if you have to go a little further than you anticipated. The main criteria are warmth, which is critical for young babies, followed by depth, the quality of the water and cleanliness. There should always be a lifeguard on duty in a public pool, but in a hotel pool or private pool where there is no lifeguard, make sure another adult who is water-confident can watch you and your baby. If you take your baby swimming in a lake, river or on a beach, that you know to be safe, the same criteria apply.

water temperature

A temperature between 31°C/88°F and 34°C/93°F is ideal to keep babies happy and comfortable. Hydrotherapy pools are usually kept around 33°C/91°F. If you only have access to a normal pool, where the water is kept at 28°C/82°F, only take babies over four months and for short sessions of about ten minutes, particularly if they are slim built. Remember that babies do not shiver when they are cold; the surplus blood from the skin is redirected to vital organs in the body, which makes their lips turn blue. Whenever you suspect that your baby may be chilled, get out and warm her up immediately. The air temperature is also important, since your baby's head and part of her body will be above the surface most of the time.

water treatment

Ozone-treated pools are preferable for babies but are relatively uncommon, as most are disinfected with chlorine. Some pools are treated with a combination of ozone and sodium hypochloride as a residual disinfectant. How chemically balanced a pool is depends a great deal on the standards of management. If, as you enter a pool, the air irritates your eyes, the chlorine levels will be too high for your baby. Test the water on your eyes before taking your baby in.

depth

Teaching pools or hydrotherapy pools in which you can stand comfortably are ideal. Depths vary from 1m/3ft to about

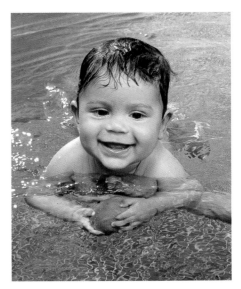

△ **Watch your baby's face and lips to make sure the temperature is comfortable for her.**

1.2m/4ft. If you are not water-confident, a shallower pool is preferable, while if you are a swimmer or are tall, greater depth is more pleasant. Variable depths have advantages and disadvantages for baby swimming, and most parents and babies adjust to the circumstances of their chosen pool.

cleanliness

Standards of hygiene are variable in public pools. The most important place to look at is the pool itself. If the filters are not operating well and the water is not absolutely clean, it is better to go to another pool if possible. The changing areas are not always kept to the highest standards, and mastering the art of changing your baby in a carrycot (carrier) or on your lap is a useful skill.

access and edges

Most training pools have constant depth and are accessible by either ladders or steps. Other shallow pools have a sloping beach-type entry on one side. Steps are preferable, as you can walk into the pool easily carrying your baby. Using a pool ladder with a baby is

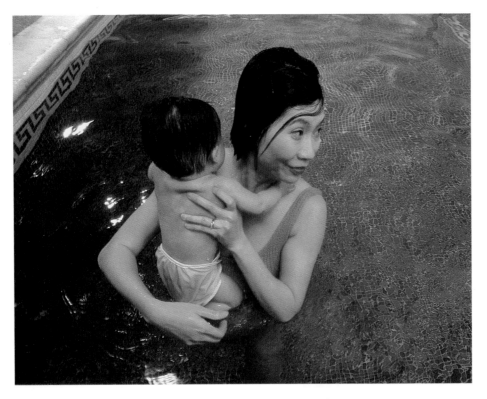

◁ **In a shallow pool, lower yourself and your baby until the water level reaches your shoulders.**

▷ Playing with floats and foam woggles (swim noodles) early on eases the transition from reflexive to voluntary movements and from your body to other forms of support.

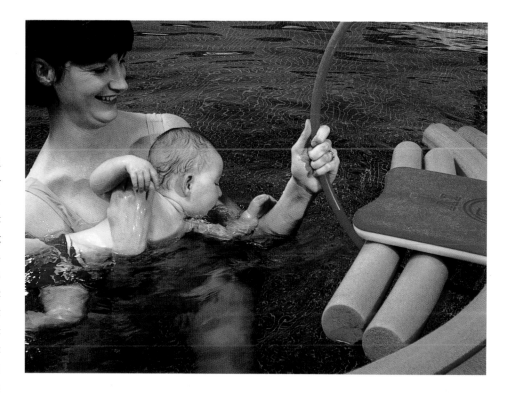

not advisable. Entering the pool safely and comfortably is the first basic skill to master before being with your baby in the water. The edges of pools vary greatly in height and build. Some have gullies that run along the pool walls; others have grab bars; others protrude slightly over the water. Grab bars are useful for older babies to hold on to, but they call for greater care when babies start jumping. Pools in which the water is not much below the level of the floor that surrounds it are preferable to pools surrounded by a raised wall where babies have to be protected from falling backwards if they sit or stand up. Adjustment to the different kinds of access and edges is made easier by adopting rules from the start about what is and is not possible. Each different entry method has a positive side that babies usually help parents to discover along the way.

atmosphere

Finally, a relaxed atmosphere, where you feel warmly welcome and encouraged to bring your baby along, is to be commended. Babies are extremely sensitive to the sounds

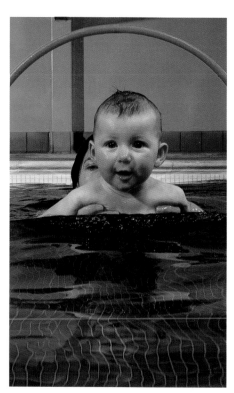

of the pool, both in and out of the water. Most babies like splashing sounds and voices in the water but tend to be put off by the high noise levels of crowded times at the pool. If possible, either take your baby to a quiet pool or use a busy pool during relatively quiet times. Remember, however, that it is the atmosphere that you create with your baby in the water that is most important.

clothing

Parents often ask what their baby should wear in the pool. Swimwear is compulsory in most public pools. Baby swimwear with a waterproof inset are now available in stores that sell nursery items. New models do not absorb water or restrict movement yet are effective in case of unpredicted accidents in the pool. They are ideal until your baby stops using diapers and can wear a swimsuit. In case you need a new swimsuit for yourself, remember that babies prefer brightly coloured ones.

Your baby's swimming equipment should also include headwear. Since babies lose a lot of heat through their heads, it is essential that you put a hat on an early swimmer before leaving the pool if it is cold outside. Sun hats are equally necessary to protect your baby's head from the sun in hot weather. If you swim outdoors, remember

◁ Keep the number of toys in the water to a minimum so as to avoid too many distractions.

that your baby is vulnerable to sunstroke while in the water.

swimming aids and toys

This book recommends that swimming aids be used as supports only, because they interfere with your baby's ability to find her balance. Armbands (arm floats), which are popular in many baby swimming schemes, are not required except in some situations that are mentioned in the various sections.

Even if you are a strong swimmer, you may want to make use of floats to relax with your baby in water. Foam woggles (swim noodles), which are increasingly popular, are versatile supports for both you and your growing baby. Two lengths, 1m/3ft and 2m/6ft, are used in this book. A standard size swimmer's foam board (kickboard) will also be useful. Models with holes for placing the hands in are preferable to plain boards.

Toys are mainly used in reinforcing skills and feeling the water. They help your baby to enjoy the water more after four months. Use one or two at most, as it is distracting for babies to be surrounded by toys in the water, particularly when they are teething. The most useful toys have proved to be small balls, squishy or not, slightly larger than a tennis ball; a plastic hoop; and for fun, a small watering can or a plastic boat. Of course, anything else that becomes your baby's favourite water toy is fine.

Start in the bath

The best way to introduce your newborn to water is in the comfort of your own home, just when it suits you and your baby. This makes the family bath the ideal place. In the bath, newborns can discover floating and feel their buoyancy, if we hold them as little as possible in the water and in a relaxed way. The family bath also has a particular atmosphere, which your baby may be familiar with since the time before birth. On the basis of thirty years' experimentation with mothers and babies in water, Russian swimming pioneer, Igor Tjarkovsky, asserts that babies' adaptation to water is actually established long before birth, hence the importance for mothers to invest time and effort to spend time in water during pregnancy. Expose your baby to the water frequently to create a continuity between fetal and newborn movement, perhaps remembering the pre-birth sensations of water surrounding his body. Make it a family bath time. It is a wonderful way to discover together your baby's experiencing of the world in a soothing, gentle, sensual way. Older children also enjoy "their" baby's bathtime and may use it to develop a close communication with him. Bath practice with your newborn anticipates the skills that will be developed later in the pool.

install yourself

Make bathtime one of the pleasurable experiences of the day, whether or not you combine it with baby massage and baby yoga. Getting your baby cleaner becomes one rather than the main purpose of bathing. Switch on your answering machine and put aside your current preoccupations. It is time to relax with your baby.

Whether your baby was born in the water or not, you can introduce him to water from day one in a large bathtub rather than a baby bath. A tub filled with 20–30cm/8–12in of water will keep both you and your baby warm and will make it possible for him to experience buoyancy.

Floating

Let your baby discover the joy of buoyancy by introducing him to water at home in the bath.

1 Get into the bath carefully and hold your baby close, facing you at first. Make sure the water level always covers at least half your baby's body. Talk to him and turn him around so that his back is loosely supported on your lap between your arms, with his legs in the water. Give your baby two or three minutes to unwind and feel the water. You can sprinkle water on your baby's tummy or back, very gently to start with. Most babies love the sensation of water trickling down on their skin.

2 Reduce the support of your hands gradually as your baby relaxes in his own way. When you feel ready, withdraw one of your hands and support your baby with one hand only, as loosely as possible. Let his head rest lightly in the palm of your hand and relax with him. This is an ideal time for singing lullabies.

3 Look at your baby and talk to him as he adjusts to all the new sensations of stretching in the water.

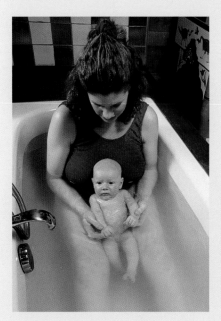

△ **Relaxing your body is a priority.**

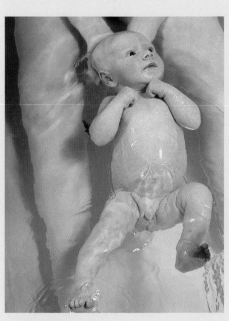

△ **Watch your baby enjoy floating.**

A comfortable water temperature is 32–33°C/90–91°F, but a range between 28°C and 34°C/82°F and 93°F suits different parents and babies. If you do not have a thermometer, the water should feel warm but not hot when you dip your elbow in. It is also important that the air temperature should be warm, about 24°C/75°F.

- Hot tubs are too warm for babies and particularly newborns unless the water is kept at 35°C/95°F or less.

- Be careful as you climb in and out of the bath while carrying your baby. Have towels at the ready next to the bath to wrap your baby up, as well as anything else that you may need.

- You may like having a non-slip mat at the bottom of the tub. Stay well clear of the hot water tap. Wet newborns can be slippery. If you are a first-time parent and handling your baby is still new to you, it is better to have someone with you at first.

the different ways your baby may respond

- If he shows you by crying that he does not enjoy this experience, take him out and cuddle him. Do not get put off if your baby's first experience in the bath is not pure bliss. Try again later, checking carefully all the variables in the environment. Some babies need cradling in the water at first; having their arms held securely along their bodies helps them to relax in the warm water.

- Relaxing in the water may make your baby kick a lot, showing you the swimming reflex. It is normal for newborns to hold their arms tight against their chest with closed fists.

- Relaxing in the water may also make your baby motionless, as if lost in a daydream, and produce smiles.

- He may stretch and start moving his legs in movements that remind you of when he was in the womb. Some newborns smile, move their heads and look relaxed. Babies' sense of touch is dominant and they take time to register all the sensations of moving freely in the water, more extensive than when they are bathed in a baby tub.

- When you have gained confidence, you may reduce the amount of support you are giving your baby's head even more. Your newborn's head is large and heavy compared with the rest of his body. Babies vary in their innate tendency to float depending on the ratio of fat tissue in their bodies and on bone density, but their head generally goes under slightly if you let go. At this stage, arm and leg movements are mostly governed by reflex behaviour.

- Let both the responses of your baby at this stage and your own feelings guide you. If you wish to remove your hand, watch your baby's reaction to having his face slightly underwater. If your baby cries, do not do this again for a couple of days. With patient practice, as your baby gets stronger week by week, he may float with just his nose and mouth above the surface. Most babies' heads need some support until a stronger leg movement can make them float. This is an excellent preparation at home until you are ready to take your baby to the pool, and it helps your newborn to discover his buoyancy from the start, long before fear has been experienced and while the gag reflex is fully operating. As long as you are with your newborn and show him your love, this can be his favourite playtime.

winding down

Clean your baby at the end of the bath and once you are out, wrap your baby securely in a large soft towel. Alternatively, breast or bottle feeding in water can be very soothing and can allow your baby to enjoy the bath for a little longer. If your baby cries, do not do it again until the next bath and take greater care to lower him gently and smoothly into the water in a continuous movement. Make sure you are relaxed before trying again. Remember that you do not have to do anything that you do not both enjoy! Even if your baby is happy, do not put his face in the water more than two or three times per bath.

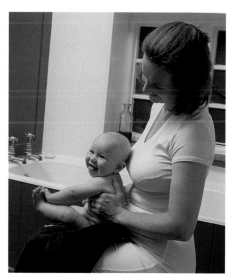

△ **After a bath, keep your baby warm by wrapping him snugly in a large, soft towel.**

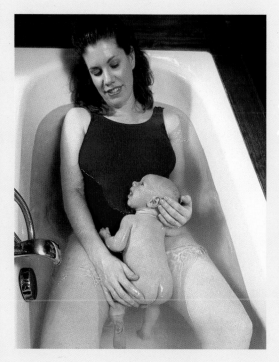

Face underwater

Changing your baby's position in the bath helps to provide different sensations and perspectives, and to exercise different muscles.

1 As you lie on your back, turn your baby face down so that he lies on your abdomen with his head just above the surface of the water. Hold him on both sides of his rib cage.

2 Then let him be freer with very gentle support only, having one hand under the base of his skull and the other reaching under his buttocks. This is a good position to gently try stimulating the diving response by lowering your baby's head face down in the water between your legs and bringing him up again on your body with your hands remaining in the same position.

3 After signalling your intent to him by making eye contact, draw him gently underwater towards you above your body using both hands. You can let the water flush your baby's face two or three times, allowing him to breathe in between. Stop if he cries. Many babies do not at all mind this preliminary version of going under and having their faces in the water.

◁ **Early submersions in the bath give your baby a head start before going to the pool.**

Getting into the pool

Even if your baby is familiar with the bath, going to the pool is a new adventure. Sharing your baby's discovery of "the big water" can trigger a wide range of emotions. What does your body language say? The more calm and confident you are, the more secure your baby will feel. Each baby needs a slightly different introduction to water. Be sensitive to particular needs and temperament and take each moment as it comes without jumping to conclusions. Some babies need more time than others to "get in" and take in all the sensations of being in the pool, while others relax immediately. Do not hurry, but be guided by your baby's response as you watch closely, yet without undue concern. Be practical: slim babies may need to wear a vest in pools that are not kept ideally warm.

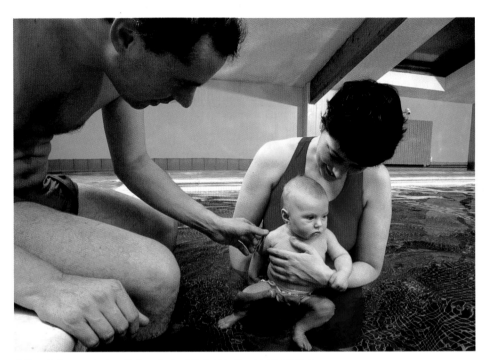

△ Your baby may look self-absorbed while taking in new sensations.

Climbing into the pool

The way you enter the pool with your baby can make a difference to her response.

1 If the pool has steps built into the side, carry your baby carefully down into the water. If there are no steps, it is best to ask someone to pass your baby to you once you are in the water for the first few times. Later, you can lower yourself into the pool with your baby. To do this, have your baby on a towel by the shallow end of the pool next to you as you sit on the edge. Slip into the water, swivelling your body so that you find yourself standing in the water facing your baby and ready to take her into your arms.

2 Once you have your baby with you in the water, hold her upright against you, either facing you or facing out, so that she adjusts to the change in environment. Make sure the water level always covers at least half of your baby's body. At the same time, relax your shoulders and your holding so that your baby experiences your support in the water rather than the feeling of being held.

3 When you are ready, lower yourself and your baby so that the water reaches your shoulders or even your neck, and rises up to your baby's neck. Keep holding your baby in as relaxed and confident a manner as possible. This gives your baby time to take in all the sensations of the water on her whole body, registering them, adjusting to them and experiencing them fully before you do anything at all. Being immersed up to the neck invites your baby to experience buoyancy from the start.

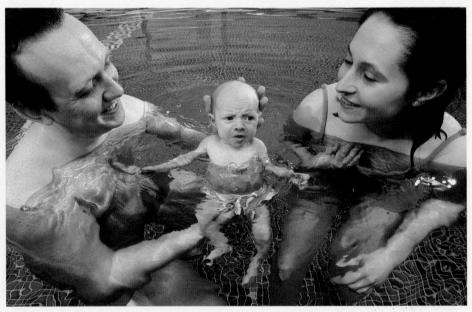

△ Hold your baby upright and make sure that the water covers at least half of her body.

In order to make the experience as happy as possible for all involved, try and eliminate anything that might inhibit the relaxation conducive to your baby feeling good in the water:

• Avoid splashing (select a quiet time at the pool or create a "baby corner").

• Have as much eye to eye communication as possible, following your baby's reactions and expressions.

• Talk reassuringly during the experience or be silent with focused attention, whichever is most appropriate.

• Resist holding your baby tightly – a secure yet unrestrictive hold, not too close to your body, is ideal.

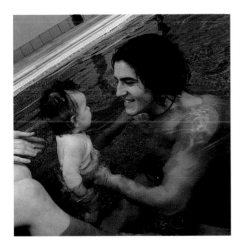

△ **Eye contact can reassure your baby that this is also an enjoyable experience for you.**

YOUR BABY MAY CRY IN THE WATER FOR VARIOUS REASONS:

• Cold (signalled by a bluish ring around her mouth).

• Tired or overstimulated (signalled by intense, unco-ordinated reflex kicking and dipping her head back in the water).

• Hungry (a small feed on the edge of the pool often helps).

• Under stress from ambient noise (increase individual attention in a quiet corner).

• Under stress from parental anxiety (play a game your baby enjoys).

• Upset by accidental dunking (older babies welcome a humorous attitude as well as comfort).

• Choking from swallowing a small amount of water (comfort and smile).

Dips and swing dips

Movement is essential when you are in the water with your baby. You need to let your baby feel secure yet unrestricted by holding her so that you offer firm yet minimal support.

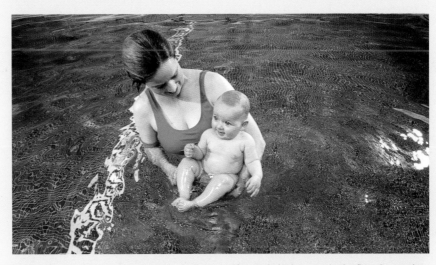

△ **Dips and swings are often the easiest way to pacify your baby in water in the first six months.**

1 Cradle your baby in an upright position in the water, holding one hand under the buttocks, supporting the head and neck with the other hand if your baby still needs head support. Dip your baby in and out of the water several times, vertically at first and then introducing a gentle rocking movement towards a reclining position.

2 If your baby enjoys this, amplify this rocking into a broader swing that dips your baby into the water with a rhythmical movement. Try different amplitudes, different rhythms and change them as your baby grows or according to her moods.

3 Be firm and daring with your movement, extending your arms without stiffening them. After gaining confidence, you can even start releasing your hand that supports your baby's head gradually at the height of the movement as your baby's spine strengthens, then placing it again under her head in the downward move of the swing.

Until your baby is about a year old, this will remain one of the most effective ways of pacifying her in the water if she has got upset. The earlier you practise it, the better, but even a baby introduced to water after six months will find this swinging movement soothing. Your baby feels the flushing of the water along her body and the resistance that it creates. For most babies, this is an enjoyable sensation. Eye contact with you, movement, rhythm and contrast between being in and out of the water are stimulating yet soothing. Some babies start lifting their heads and kicking vigorously with this movement; others relax with it. What your baby does today will change as she grows.

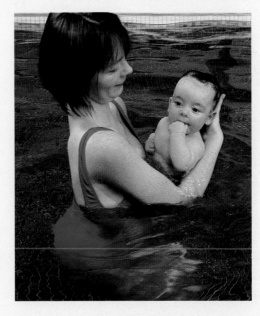

▷ **As you enter the pool with your baby, small dips in synchrony allow you to lower yourselves in the water while remaining close.**

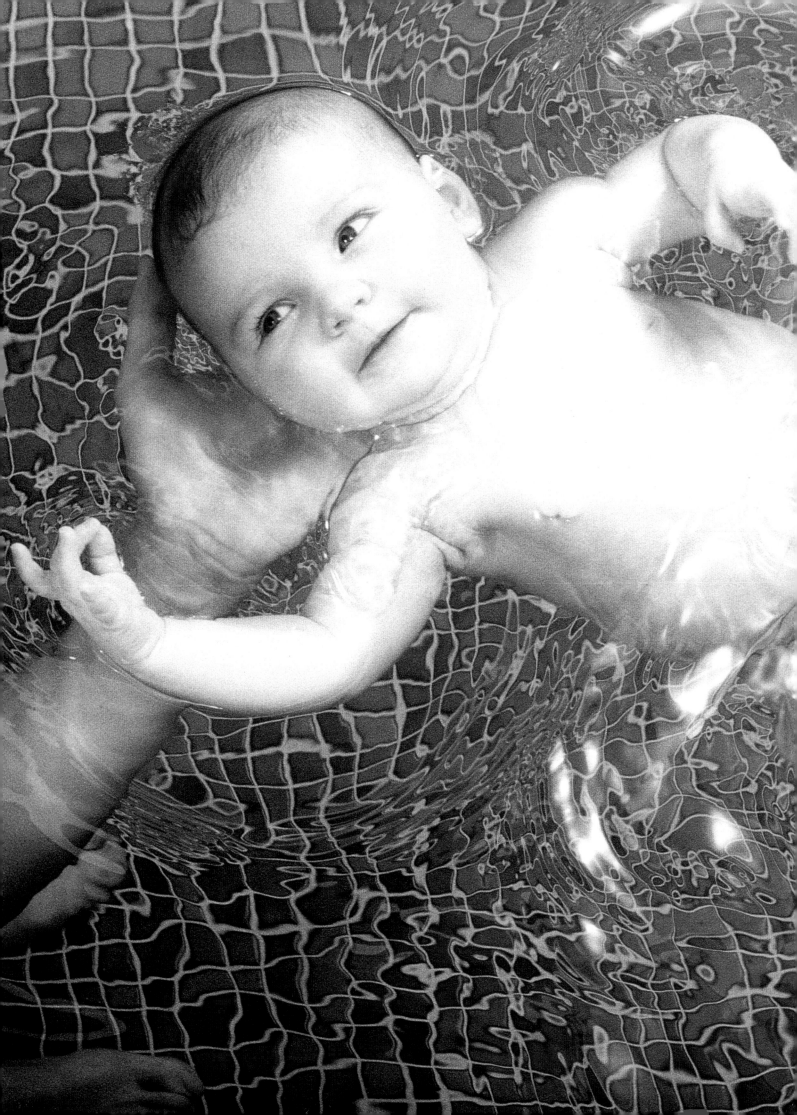

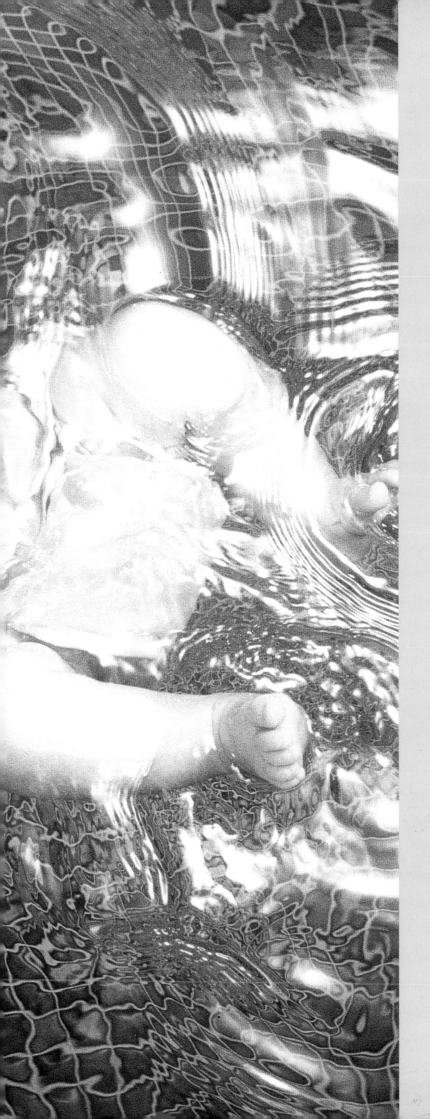

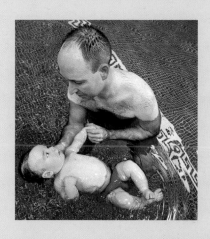

floating

The experience of floating is one that comes naturally to young babies and gives them great pleasure. It allows a newborn to experience water with all his senses in close communication with you, the supporting parent. The security that your baby feels gently floating on your hand, and the eye contact and intimacy between you will strengthen your bond and confirm your mutual love.

Back float

After a few dips and swing dips, you are ready to practise the "floating hold" – that is, to hold your baby as little as possible to encourage her to float on her back. It is supremely important to encourage a correct back position from the start as a foundation for future swimming. The back float presented here, in which support under the baby's head is gradually removed, tends to stimulate babies' kicking in a good body alignment and prepares them to float effortlessly as toddlers. A small minority of babies with strong kicking spontaneously progress from back float to unaided swimming on their backs.

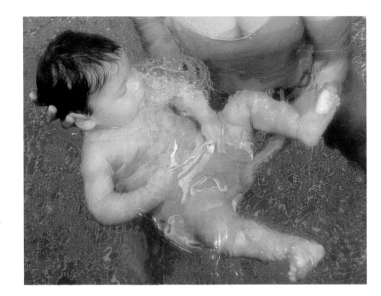

◁ **From swing dips, remove the hand that is supporting your baby's buttocks. This allows her to tip back into a floating position.**

Slowly letting go

Teaching your baby to float on her back is a slow and gentle process.

1 When your baby reaches the reclined position of the dip in the water, all you need to do to "float" her is to remove your hand that supports her buttocks, keeping a supporting hand under her head. This may not feel very secure to you at first, so you may want to bring your other hand up to cradle your baby's head. Try not to support your baby's head with one hand and her back with the other, since this does not give her the freedom to float.

2 For a good horizontal alignment, the level of the water should reach just above your baby's ears. Try to keep your baby's head in line with her body. Make sure that your hands under her head remain relaxed and open with soft palms holding your baby's skull. Support her as lightly as possible, relaxing your arms and shoulders. Chubby babies float more easily than slim babies, who may need to be held more. Rocking your baby gently at first may help her relax more, making floating easier.

3 After a few sessions, remove the support of your hands gradually until one finger is left under your baby's head. If your baby's head control is not yet secure, as you let go with the supporting hand her head will tend to flop backwards, causing her face to be covered by water. While some babies do not seem to mind at all and may kick or not, others take in water and choke, which may cause them to make frantic arm and leg reflex movements. If this happens, pick up your baby gently and cuddle her. Try again when her neck is stronger.

4 As babies' reflexive kicks get stronger, the water level will be around their faces, sometimes up to their eyes and mouths, but no longer covering their noses so that they can continue to breathe. As babies kick and stay up, the association between the two strengthens. Talk to your baby directly above her face and click your fingers to help keep her head raised, which she will tend to do automatically around six months. For a baby over four months you can also hold a familiar colourful toy. Stop as soon as your baby gets tired; lift her up smoothly, cuddle and praise her.

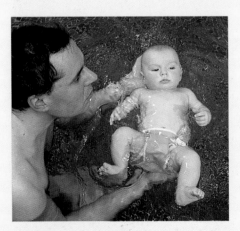

△ **Relax as you hold your baby.**

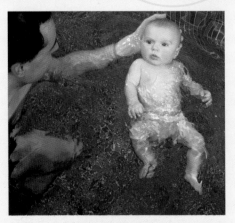

△ **Gradually remove your "seat hand".**

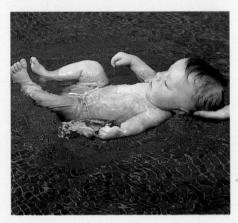

△ **The water level should be just above the ears.**

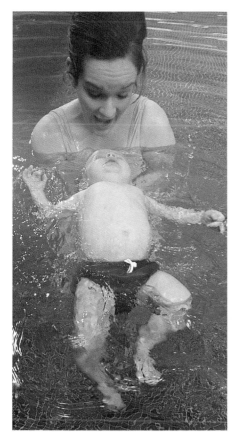

△ Some babies seek eye contact and love to "talk" while they float.

Trying to sit up while in the back floating position is a natural reaction for babies over five months, due to the "righting reflex" and a better head control. If your baby resists lying back and wants to keep her head upright, do not use force. Focus on front holding for a few weeks and then try again. Also, keep practising turning in the "safety position" and float your baby with her front on your chest. Let this process follow its course but keep trying back float again at regular intervals. Resistance to floating can last for a couple of months while babies master neck control, after which they revert to floating again. Do not force a baby who resists being on her back as there are so many other skills that can be developed wihout her needing to be on her back. If your baby has been floating happily before, she will resume floating easily later on. An older baby or toddler may resist the back float and discover the sensation of floating in a different way. Some babies progress spontaneously from reflexive kicking to an early form of backstroke. If your baby likes back floats, encourage this practice as a survival skill before your baby develops the strength to swim prone.

active floating

While the righting reflex and greater neck and head control together cause babies to lift their heads as early as four months and to try and roll to a prone position, active floating is a way to continue encouraging your baby to enjoy back floats in preparation for swimming on her back. In *Birthlight* classes, parents have found that their babies particularly enjoyed the following ways of active floating; perhaps you can find others.

float swap

Practise sending your baby to someone else for floating. Support your baby's back while the other person supports the head in their hands. Draw your floating baby towards you, say hello and gently send her back, releasing your hand when her head is supported by the other person again, who then says hello from above.

walk-float

Walking backwards in the water creates a current that helps your baby's legs stay afloat, particularly in the case of an older baby. If your baby moves vigorously in a happy way as you walk-float, gradually remove your hand or hands from under her head, allowing her to float unaided. Keep your hands in the water just under her head and support it again if it starts to sink. You can also raise your baby's head a little for breathing at close intervals, which is one way of making your baby experience the contrast between breathing on the surface and "closing" for later swimming.

snake-float, bob-float

Spice up the walk-float with a zig-zag movement or a figure of eight. Older babies enjoy this more rapid movement and usually do not resist it even though they refuse to do plain back float. You can make this movement even more exciting by including an up and down rolling movement besides the circular ones, bobbing your floating baby along.

tug-float

If you are a confident swimmer, take your floating baby, or even newborn, for a little swim round the pool, supporting the back of her head with one hand while you swim on your back, tugging her by your side. This introduces greater movement and gives your baby different sensations altogether. Trailing your floating baby in this way is much easier than it sounds. You are swimming together freely, only bound by the palm of one hand, yet safe, as you can readily lower your legs to stand in the pool without ceasing to support your baby.

▽ In "active floating", babies experience the swift movement of water along their bodies.

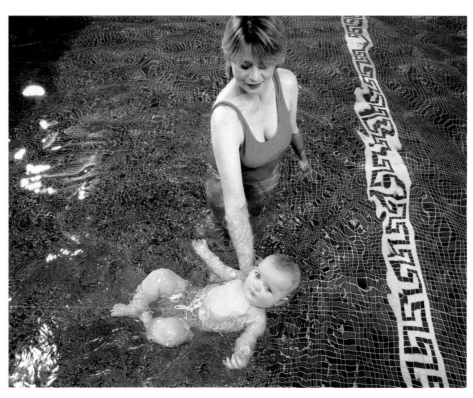

The spirit of floating

Whether or not babies actually remember the sensations of being in the womb, the powerful effects of water on the human psyche extend to newborns. Life began in the ocean, and mythologies across the world depict human evolution in relation to water. Floating and diving are two ways of being in water that modify aspects of our physiology in measurable ways. The development of waterbirthing publicized the relaxing effect of water during labour for mothers and possibly for their babies. Supporting babies to float continues what they may have experienced if their mothers practised "floating relaxation" during pregnancy. If, however, you are not familiar with floating and you are just introducing your baby to water, it is worth taking time to follow your baby's experience of floating and also to relax and float with him in the water. This is ideally practised with your spouse or partner or with a friend who can help you get comfortable with your baby and watch both of you as you float together.

floating relaxed

As you support your baby's head and watch him stretch and relax in the water, you are likely to enjoy a very special kind of intimacy mediated by water. This can be started in the bath and expanded in the pool. Once you are supporting your baby

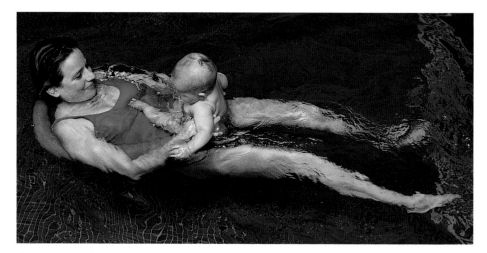

△ Foam woggles (swim noodles) make it possible for less confident parents to float with their babies.

with his ears in water and just his face out, try and remain steady to keep the water level constant, relaxing in your supporting position. While at first you encourage splashing and kicking when supporting your baby for floating, you can also use this position for relaxing with your baby. Older babies that arch backward or roll to the side, which causes their heads to submerge, or very active young babies, may find this just as challenging as kicking is to very calm babies. Babies who cry in the back position can be cradled in a semi-sitting position, which allows them to enjoy being in the water while staying in your arms.

Once you are settled, let your baby find his own space in the water, experiencing unboundedness and freedom of movement. Maintain eye contact and keep talking to your baby. Some babies get absorbed in a deep daydream of their own; in this case, do not force eye contact if your baby looks away happily. Try to avoid interfering stimuli such as bright lights on the pool ceiling above your baby's face. Babies of all ages experiment with stretching according to their stage of development. It is important not to be in a hurry and to allow your baby the time that he needs for this experience. This can be as much as a few minutes, uninterrupted. Let your baby signal the end of floating to you. Some

babies like doing it for longer than others and have it as their favourite activity while others prefer to be on their front early on.

joint floating relaxation with your baby

This is particularly beneficial for new fathers, although mothers should practise it in the same way and both parents can take turns in the pool. Sometimes it is hard for a new mother to entrust her newborn to the father but this is also part of the challenge. Adults who need to feel very secure while floating can either use a foam board (kickboard) under their lower back or a couple of foam woggles to support themselves as they lower their bodies in the

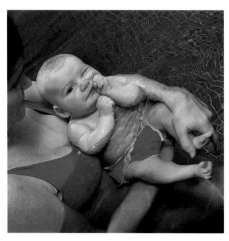

△ Babies enjoy the difference between being held in water and floating with their parents.

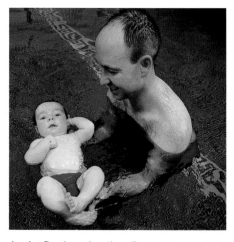

△ Joint floating relaxation allows new parents to bond with their babies in the water.

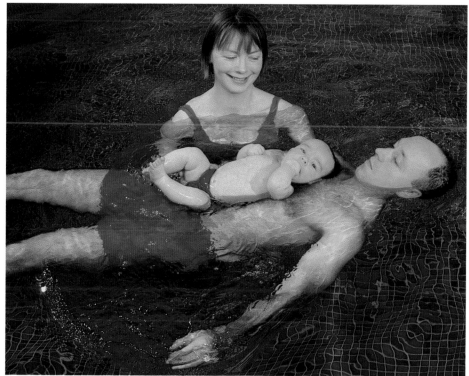

◁ Allowing your baby to be unrestrained on your floating body (here supported by a board under the lower back) adds to the experience of joint relaxation. It is helpful to have mother keeping watch.

water. The exchange that takes place when both parents are involved is threefold, between the baby, the parent who supports and floats the baby and between the watching parent and the baby.

Floating brings about positive associations with pleasure, closeness and security. Taking time to float allows parents to enjoy relaxing with their babies in water rather than rushing into swimming exercises geared towards achievement. For babies, floating with parents creates a lasting association between water and wellbeing as well as a foundation for learning to swim from inborn reflexes and free movement. Babies who experience floating relaxation with their parents appear both calm and alert.

therapy floating

In the late 1960s, Tjarkovsky became interested in the benefits of swimming for babies after helping his underweight, sick, premature daughter to a rapid recovery by holding her in water every day. His results with the babies of athletes in the former Soviet Union have been impressive, but undermined by his forceful dipping of babies underwater, which was contested in other countries. Without intense immersion, which may be traumatic to babies, it is possible to learn from Tjarkovsky's pioneering discoveries about the therapeutic effects of water on early

development, more particularly when babies have been born with a particular condition or handicap that needs a different approach.

Having a baby who is different from the norm is a challenge for any parent. Floating can be practised with any baby, once your doctor has confirmed that it is safe to take him to the pool, and the benefits are not only emotional but can also be therapeutic. Babies who have had a traumatic birth, spent time in an incubator or have undergone interventions during and after

birth may be less readily happy in the water than others. If your baby screams in the bath and nothing seems to help, sit with him in a very shallow bath, sprinkling water on your body at first. Gradually move on to sitting your baby against you in the shallow water and sprinkling his feet and legs. Feeding your baby in the bath, if possible, helps this transition. With patience, you will progress towards floating and seeing your baby enjoy the sensations of water on her body.

The healing properties of the water are partly due to the fact that it enables a different form of communication. This is often a deep intuitive silent contact that is not mediated directly by words. The water acts as a medium in which it is easier to enjoy just being, not only because it frees our bodies, but also because it surrounds us. Babies with Down's syndrome do remarkably well in water and can become early swimmers. Floating, perhaps with a vest at first if your baby dislikes being undressed, also allows tense babies to gradually relax to the point of opening their arms freely in their own time.

CASE STUDY: PENNY AND CHAD

Taking my son, Chad, with all his breathing difficulties into the water for the very first time was quite a frightening prospect, and I was rather apprehensive. But I adore the water and could understand Françoise's reasoning for this therapy. Chad was fretful at first, but Françoise showed me how to float with Chad, and it was a lovely feeling to be so close to him in the water. He was on my chest and gradually I found the confidence to let go

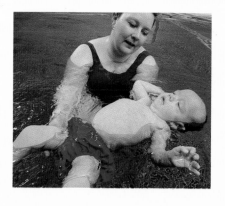

of him, his little head resting under my chin. I soon realized, to my amazement, that he had relaxed completely, and fallen asleep. He was totally at peace and sound asleep as I swam backstroke up and down the pool. He was still aware of the water, as he turned his head away from the ripples as they touched his face, but still totally relaxed. I put my hand on his chest to feel him "purring" contentedly like a cat. It was amazing, and when I lifted Chad out of the water, he awoke immediately and was very cross. He did not want to be disturbed. I was totally elated and chatted non-stop to my mother about it, while Chad slept soundly all the way home.

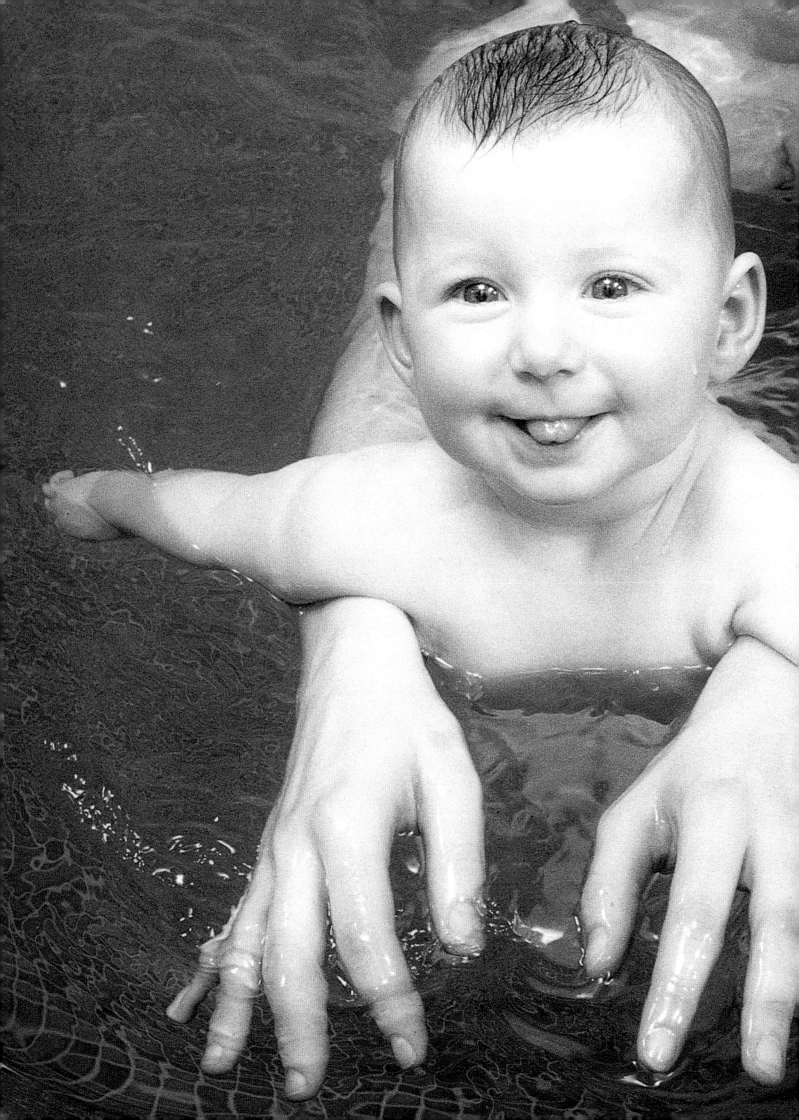

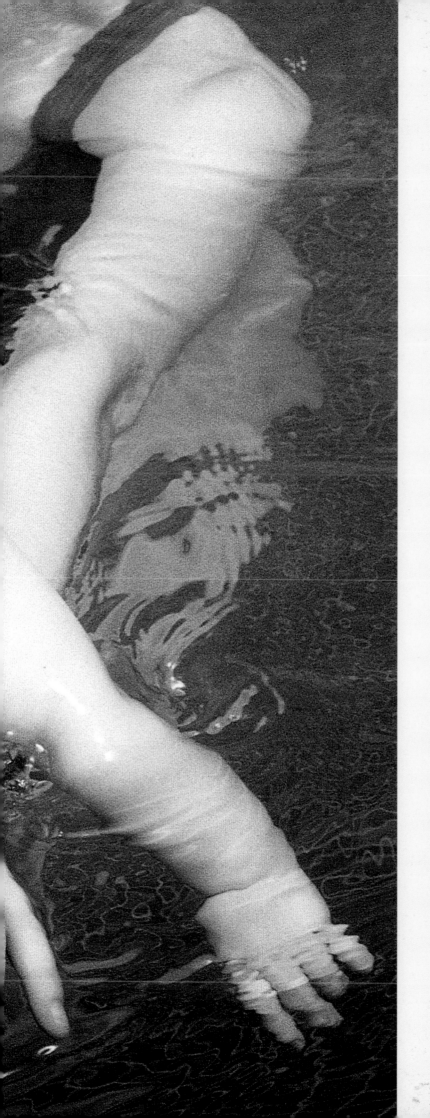

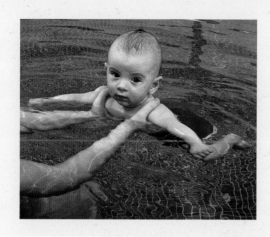

holding
for
swimming

These exercises will show you different ways of holding your baby in the water as early swimming reflexes gradually become deliberate movements. You should not rush these exercises. They are the foundation of future unaided swimming. Repeat them each week so that skills can be consolidated in all different positions. As your baby's confidence grows, encourage independence but, at the same time, always make sure that your baby feels safe and secure.

Safety position

This is a way of holding your baby facing away from you that gives maximum freedom to move and prepares your baby for swimming on his front. The safety position, as its name indicates, is a very secure base that allows many variations that, in turn, allow your baby to venture away from your arms and feel comfortable while being held less and less. This position also seems to be one that stimulates most swimming reflexes in your baby, particularly vigorous kicks. It provides a comfortable starting point for launching your baby forward, above or underwater, in baby dives. It can be used as your basic holding position in the water, from birth throughout your baby's first year. If you need to change or adjust the way you are holding your baby in the safety position, an easy way of doing so is to lift one of your knees in the water and sit your baby on it for a moment.

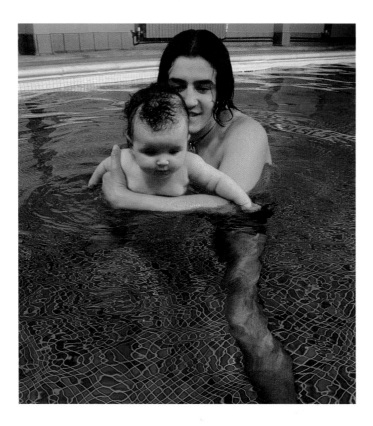

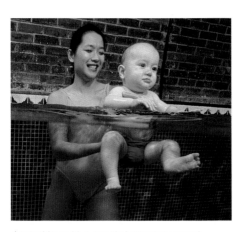

◁ In the safety position, your strong hand supports your baby's seat while your other arm extends across her chest to keep her head above water.

Safety hold

The "safety hold" is the most basic way to hold your baby in water so as to encourage movement. It allows you to be active too, gradually releasing one of your hands and feeling freer with your baby in the water.

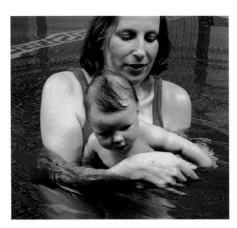

△ **1** As you stand in the water, support your baby facing away from you with one outstretched arm across his chest. Your hand extends under his arm. For additional safety, you may grip your baby's arm between your thumb and index finger, but this is not necessary unless you need it for your reassurance.

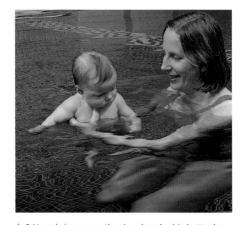

△ **2** Now, bring your other hand under his buttocks. Use your strong hand (right if you are right-handed) as your "seat hand" and the other to support your baby's chest. He should now be leaning forward on your outstretched arm while your other hand can move him more or less upright, closer to your body or further away from you. Try these various movements, relaxing your shoulders more and more. As you gain confidence, hold your baby further away from your body.

△ **3** In this position, your baby tends to propel himself forward, often with vigorous kicks. If he does not, bob gently up and down, raising him a little above the surface and lowering again as upright as possible. Sooner or later, he will start throwing his legs together, pulling them up and extending them in turn, the movement that makes very young babies look as though they are truly swimming.

▷ Most babies love rolling movements. By rolling your baby from a safety hold on to a back-float position, you can say hello and have a cuddle, or take off in backstroke with him.

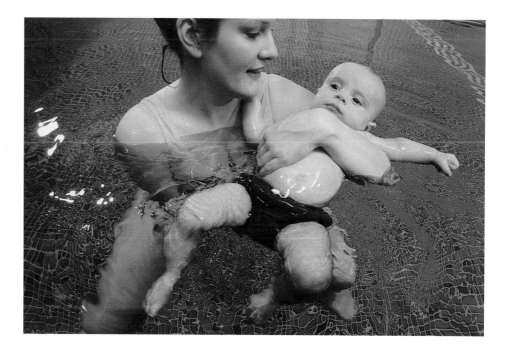

various holding positions

Once you are comfortable with this holding position, you can use many variations of it. Here are only a few of those that you may discover as you spend time in water with your baby.

rolling to float

It is easy to move from the safety position to a cradling back float by rolling your baby gently along your outstretched arm, using your seat hand for direction, so that his head comes to rest on the inside of your elbow. He is now floating with his head comfortably on your arm. Most babies like the sensation of turning over and rolling. You can then unroll him back into the safety position when you are both ready. This can be practised even with older babies who lift their heads. It can also be done as a cuddly game to create closeness when needed during your session. You can also use your seat hand to facilitate rolling.

arm support only

Once your shoulders are relaxed in the safety position, you can hold your baby loosely with one arm across his chest. When your baby starts consciously reaching for toys, use a ball to stimulate movement of his legs and later of his arms. You may be surprised at his kicking and stretching forward to the ball. This is also a preparation for using a foam woggle, instead of your arm as a support later on during your baby's transition to independent swimming.

chest hold

Soon you will no longer need to extend your arm right around your baby's chest – holding your hand quite loosely will provide effective support as well as give your baby increasing freedom. Practise resting his chest on your hand only, gradually removing your seat hand. Your baby will soon become accustomed to this position if your hand is firm and stable. This is a good preparation for baby surf.

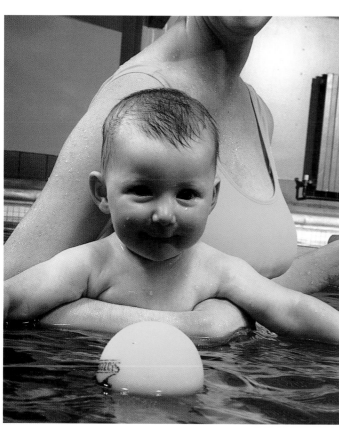

△ **Arm support only is a preparation for using a foam woggle (swim noodle).**

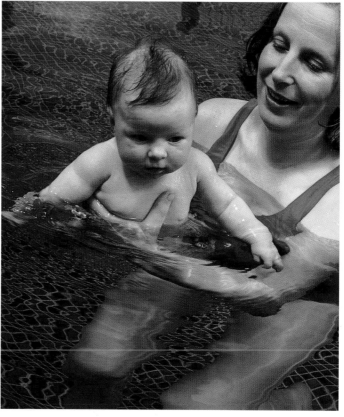

△ **Hand support under the chest is a preparation for baby surf.**

Opening the safety position

After a few weeks, you may feel relaxed enough to open the safety position and support your baby with one hand only, placing it across or under her chest. This allows you to reduce your support gradually so that your baby finds her own buoyancy and can move both her legs and arms. Think of giving her the minimum support she needs to remain on her front on the water surface. She will inevitably have her face in the water sometimes, but resting on your arm is a source of security that should make accidental dunking tolerable. If your baby swallows water or chokes, stop and comfort her. This is also a suitable position to introduce your baby to duckling dives and to practise front surf.

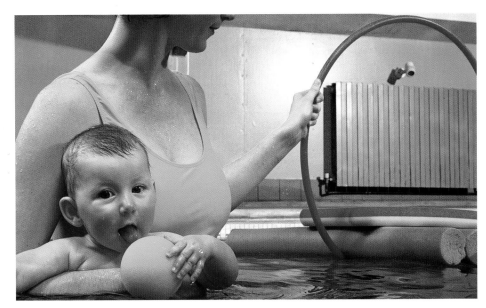

△ A relaxed safety hold is useful when you need to use your other hand or change position.

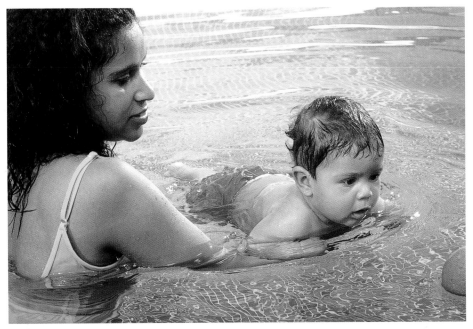

△ In the open safety position, your baby will make a circular movement traced by your opening arm.

how to do it

Supporting your baby with one arm, lower her so that her face is just above the surface of the water and extend your arm out in a wide semicircle. Turn around to make another circle, and another. This takes your baby away from your body and gets her used to being held as little as possible for swimming. Relax your arm and let your baby lean on it as little as possible. After six months, a ball gives an incentive to your baby to propel herself forward more. A parent can also be a very attractive target – older babies love playing chase games. These various ploys may activate the transition from reflexive to deliberate kicking.

The challenge is to have your baby steady on your relaxed arm. Once this has been achieved, you will be able to substitute a foam woggle (swim noodle) for your arm.

encouraging kicking

The transition to deliberate kicking is smooth if your baby can feel relaxed and secure in the water and associates leg movements with effectively propelling herself forward towards an attractive target. If you start with an older baby who has lost the swimming reflex, the first task is to move

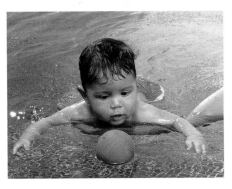

△ Balls encourage arm movements.

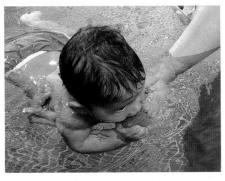

△ Let your baby catch the ball some of the time.

▷ With practice, parents or friends can pass on a baby to each other in the opened safety position. Make sure your baby's face remains above the surface if she tends to swallow water.

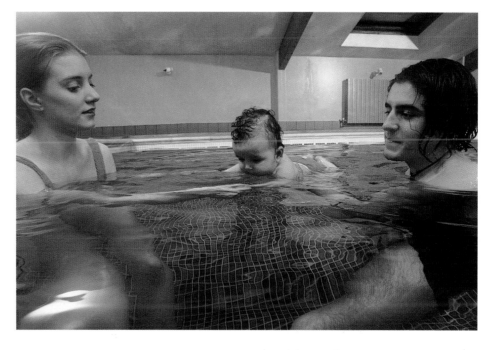

your baby in the water before you encourage kicking. Not all babies kick spontaneously. Do not be alarmed if your child is relaxed but shows no desire for kicking.

Kicking can also be done by another person moving your baby's legs while you hold her on her front or back. If you are on your own, you can move your baby's legs with your free hand in the open safety position. When you see your baby kick spontaneously or when you move your baby's legs up and down, reinforce the association by saying "kick, kick" so that your baby can be reminded of kicking more in the different positions with less and less support. Each baby will kick in a different way: some with a cycling movement;

others with a frog kick, using both legs at once; others asymmetrically; others using the various forms of kicking in succession or together in one session. Do not try and shape your baby's kicking until she can swim unaided.

◁ Lifting your baby above water with your "seat hand" while your other hand supports her chest stimulates vigorous kicking.

Baby-swimming pioneers around the world are in agreement that young children are generally not capable of consciously refining their kicks until the age of two, usually over.

flip flops

An open version of rolling to float is known as flip flops. You are now shifting support from your baby's chest to her back with one hand, trying to widen the gap between your hands with practice. Your baby goes from a prone position to a back-floating position alternately in a movement that you can make rhythmical and more lively as your baby grows stronger.

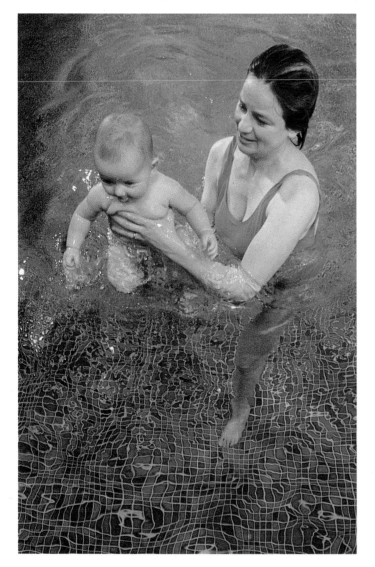

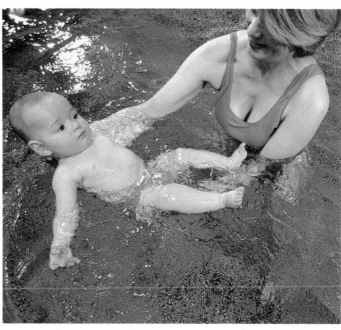

△ Flip flops give your baby a first taste of the contrast between front crawl and backstroke.

Seat hold games

Babies enjoy the experiences of being in water. They are soon keen to socialize and interact with other babies and adults, sometimes more readily than on dry land. Babies love water games in which they participate closely with their parents. The following two games are based on the "safety position" but with your "seat hand", the hand that supports your baby's buttocks, given priority. The aim is progressively to increase the strength of babies' backs, stimulate their reflexive kicking and provide enjoyable dynamic movements in the company of other adults and babies.

seat hold

Once you are comfortable with the basic safety position, you can rely mainly on your strong hand for a seat hold in which your baby balances on your seat hand in the

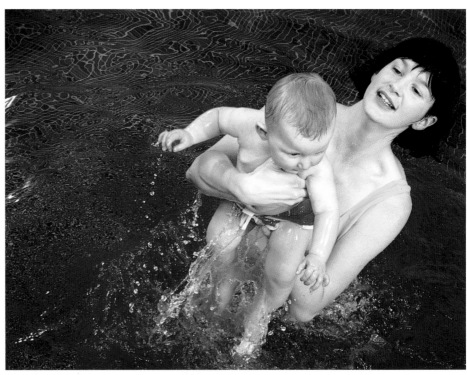

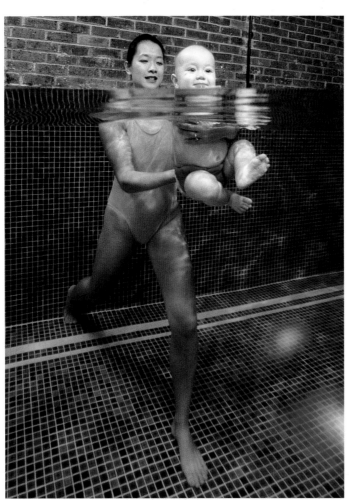

▷ Using both buoyancy and your baby's growing strength, hold him upright in a sitting position with just his head above water. Catch him with your other hand if you lose his balance.

△ Babies have a strong sense of rhythm. As soon as they are familiar with the pool, games that involve to and fro movements, away from you and back to you, are greatly enjoyed.

water, with only his head above the surface. This way of holding is popular in Russian baby water-training programmes. It develops babies' back muscles and triggers the kicking swimming reflex to an even greater extent than the safety position. It takes some practice to achieve a steady balance, but the deeper you and your baby are in the water, the easier it is to start balancing. The activity of your baby's back muscles may surprise you in this movement.

seat throws

With some practice, you can use the seat hold to lift your baby above the water surface with remarkably little effort, since your baby can hold himself upright with his spinal muscles. Your other arm extends in front of your baby to offer a fender so that he does not fall forward into the pool, or at least not just yet. At first, you are likely to do these

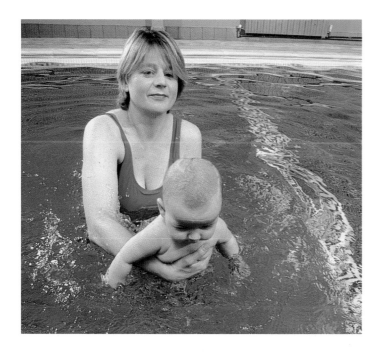

◁ Seat throws are a good exercise for mothers too. Adjust your safety position, encouraging your baby's kicking with small dips ...

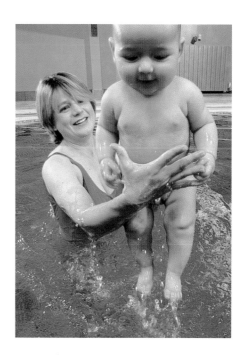

▷ ... and when you are both ready, standing firmly, lift your baby up and lower him again in to the water, close to your body.

▷ Babies enjoy water parties very early in life. Standing at about an arm's length from other parents and babies, get ready to "whoosh".

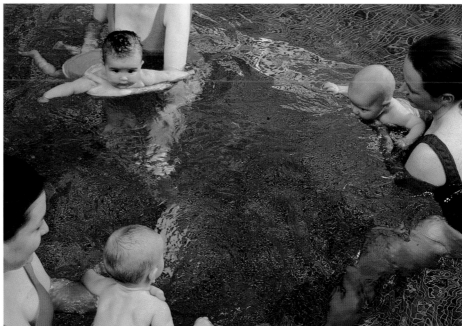

lifts quite close to your body; as you gain confidence, lifts become higher and more dynamic. It is then best to have a strong launching position with one foot forward, bending your knee to create a secure base. You will soon become able to lift your baby up and ahead of you above the water, dipping him and bringing him back towards you in the water before starting again. Do these throws gently with young babies, gradually increasing the height as your baby grows. Always draw him back into the water.

whooshing

This is basically a seat throw directed towards another or other babies in the pool. "Whoosh" is the sound that emerged spontaneously in the *Birthlight* classes to accompany this popular movement, which delights everyone involved. Babies seem to enjoy immensely the alternate closeness and distance with other little people while being held securely by a parent. "Whoosh" as long as the strength of your arms allows, lifting your baby as he gets near to his little friends, with a synchronized movement of each parent–and–baby pair.

▷ "Whooshing", particularly with matching sounds and actions, can be a highlight of your regular session at the pool with friends and their babies.

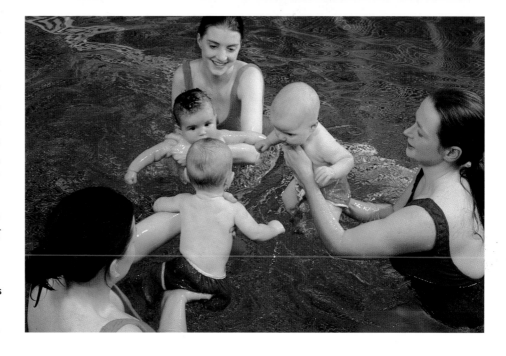

Front holding

Front holding allows you to keep eye contact with your baby as you hold her securely under her arms. It is a good point of departure for future jumping, for immersion and submersion, for the transition to swimming and to show your baby how to blow out into the water from six months onwards. However, it allows your baby less freedom of movement than the previous safety position, and does not give as much support to babies under four months. Front holding can soon be replaced by "front surf" to give your baby a good alignment in swimming prone.

front safe holding

Hold your baby facing you with your hands under her armpits; your thumbs are raised above her shoulders while your index fingers support her arms. In this position, which should only be used on babies with sufficient head control, pull her forward for a kiss and push her back again a few times so that she feels the movement of the water. You should also be standing in the water with only your head above the surface so that your movements are as much in the water as possible. Keep your shoulders relaxed.

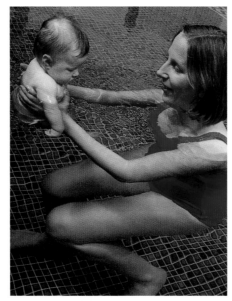

△ It may take from one to ten sessions for a baby to imitate blowing.

bubble blowing

It is not easy for infants to learn bubble blowing because the sucking reflex prevails until about six months. It means exhaling through the mouth, which is a new skill, since nearly all babies breathe through their noses. Introduce this new sensation of blowing with an element of fun, by blowing bubbles and spitting out water in front of

your baby, making noisy bubbles, and spurting like a horse. Showing your baby how to blow may take a number of sessions until your baby is able to switch from sucking to blowing. The more you have shown her how to do it in the water, the easier she will do it once she gets the gist of it. Show your baby how to spit out water by making a little spurt towards her. Older babies find this very funny and will practise intensely to imitate.

front glide

Hold your baby facing you and so that her face is just above the surface. Signal to her to take a breath, particularly if she is over six months, and draw her towards you, face down in the water, picking her up close to your body. If she cries, you are then ready to comfort her. If she is happy, hold her at arms' length and, with a pull towards you, let her come to you under the surface before picking her up gently close to your body again. This can be one of the ways of starting to swim if your baby moves vigorously to reach you. You can then increase the distance gradually from a few centimetres/inches to 2 m/6 ft in a few weeks.

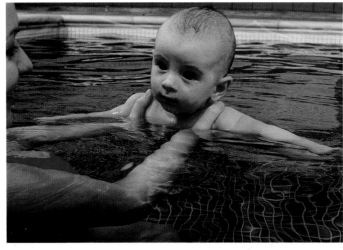

△ Front holding is most effective if your face and your baby's face are on the same level, just above the water.

▷ Front holding leads rapidly to movement, drawing your baby forward in a "front glide" and gently pushing her back again.

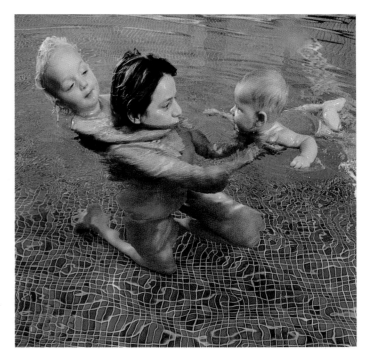

▷ Holding your baby under the arms or just under the chin prepares her for a good alignment of the body in future unaided swimming.

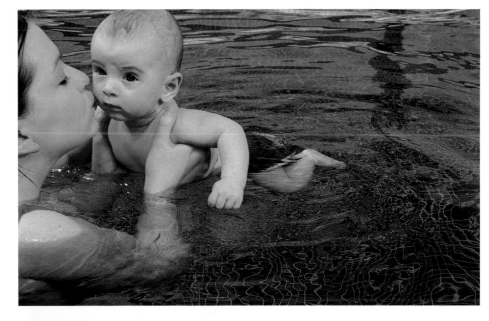

With babies up to four months, support under the chin is preferable to support under the arms so that their mouths stay just above water. You can hold your baby's chin in your two hands making a V-shape or, if she is quite buoyant, use only one hand. If your newborn is happy when her face goes underwater, you can also draw her towards you in this way, picking her up gently by putting your other hand under her buttocks in a seat lift to bring her close to your body.

front surf

Holding your baby with one of your hands under her chest in front surf is suitable for all babies from birth throughout the first year. For this way of front holding, you need to be relaxed and not mind the occasional tumble into the water. This gives your baby the maximum posssibility of movement in a prone position. Adjust your hand so that your baby has the best possible alignment while keeping her mouth and nose just above the surface. Some babies do not mind having their faces in the water now and

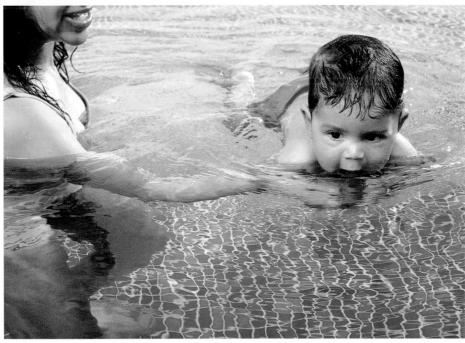

▷ Your baby can move freely with your hand supporting only her chest, as in front surfing.

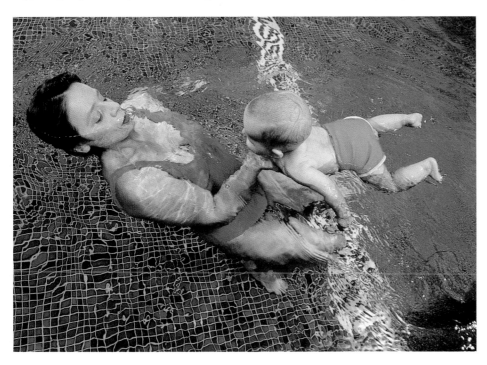

then; others dislike this intensely. Surf your baby around you with as much movement as possible, forwards and sideways. This is more advanced than opening the safety position, as your baby is supported on only one point of her body and has free arms.

swim baby tug

If you are a confident swimmer and you can front surf your baby comfortably, why not take off on your back, dragging her along with your hand under her chest along the pool? The more rapidly you swim, the more your baby is buoyant and active.

◁ Tugging your baby along in "front surf" is not difficult once you feel your baby's buoyancy.

Little harbour

The idea is to encourage the baby to hold on rather than you holding him; let him find his freedom yet offer him adequate support in the water. This position has been named the "little harbour" in *Birthlight* baby classes because you are making a harbour with your arms that your baby can launch from and can come back to safely. This can also lead your baby to "pulling" with his arms voluntarily when the swimming reflex subsides.

establishing the position

Standing in the pool with the water up to chest level, extend your arms under your baby's arms so that he is supported upright in the water, facing away from you. Your baby may try and hold your wrists, which is fine, although the little harbour position encourages babies to keep their arms relaxed or even floppy. Keep your shoulders relaxed, giving a loose support to your baby. You can introduce movement within the safety of the little harbour: making waves,

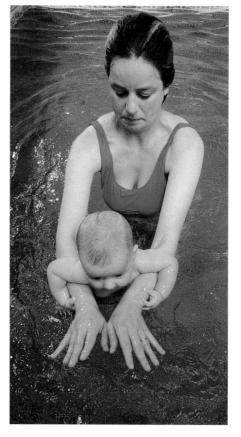

◁ **At first, your baby may grip your extended arms as you make a little harbour for him.**

bobbing, swinging, circling with your parallel arms supporting your baby, and perhaps other movements you can discover too.

little harbour splashing

Splashing in front of babies is a good way of encouraging arm movement as they soon try to imitate you – if not immediately. Babies differ a great deal about splashing and it is important to respond to your baby's particular inclination at any stage.

Start with very gentle splashing with your fingers for very young babies, until they start joining in with you. The freer your baby is with having his face in water, the more he usually enjoys splashing. Discourage too much splashing, as it is wasted energy as far as swimming is concerned, and encourage true propelling arm movements. "Pulling" is the arm movement that babies

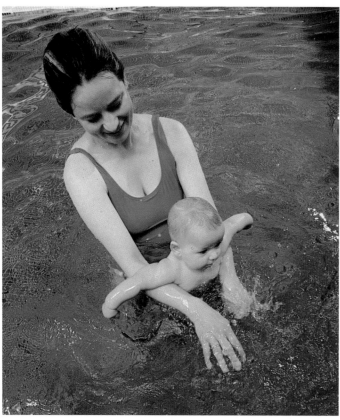

△ **As your baby gets confident, he opens his arms and kicks while you splash.**

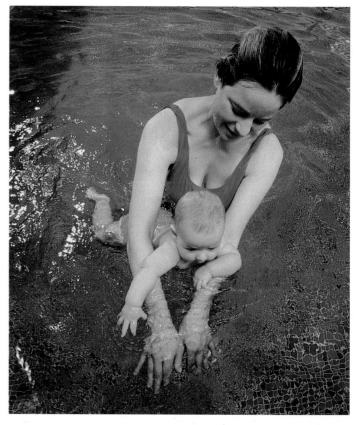

△ **Movements of your arms prepare your baby for future "pulling" with his arms.**

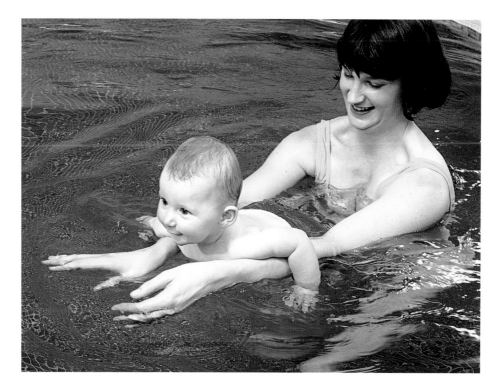

▷ In the little harbour, babies enjoy being propelled forward on their front and then dragged towards you on their backs.

first use to propel themselves, either with both arms symmetrically or with alternate arms as paddling. In the little harbour, the progression is from the parent splashing to baby splashing to pulling. It is more effective if your baby's shoulders can be kept close to or under the surface of the water. Encourage asymmetrical front crawl movements of your baby's shoulders by moving your arms alternately. You are now inviting your baby to make use of his arms for pulling in the water when he starts swimming. This arm movement will be your baby's main source of propulsion together with the leg movement in the early stages of unaided swimming, making surfacing to breathe possible.

games in the little harbour

From the stable, little harbour position, you can launch your baby forward with your arms, still supporting his arms, so that he reaches a little friend. You can also make a circling movement, in the opposite direction to a friend, so that the babies meet again and again when the circles bring them together. Babies like going back and forth between their parents too. While you launch out your baby, the other parent is ready to receive him in a front holding position and can then send him back to you again out of the little harbour. Launching-out games also give your baby an important safety skill that progressively trains him to hold on to a support in the water.

Babies over five months also like to reach out for a toy. With older babies, it is fun to play mini-water-polo games.

▽ Little friends – here a twin – are ideal incentives to move to while in the safety of the little harbour.

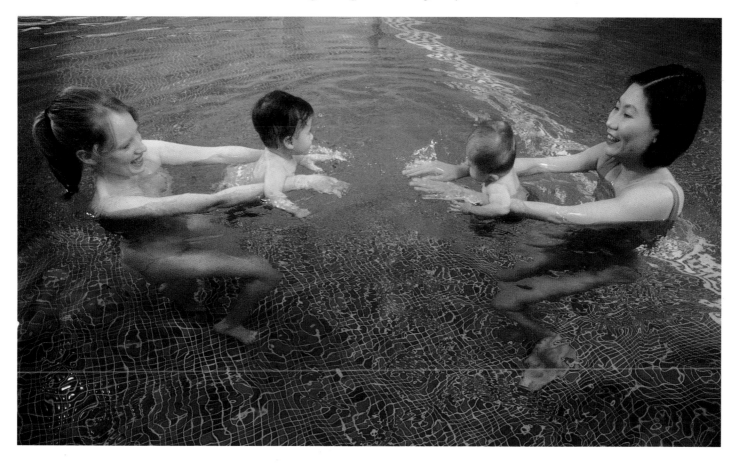

Figures of eight

This is the most dynamic of the exercises in which you stimulate your baby's movement on the surface of the water while you stand in the pool. Starting with an opening of the little harbour, you make full use of your baby's acquired buoyancy to shift her from front to back positions, offering minimal support by letting her hold your hands. These movements make figures of eight in the water. They help your baby to move on to being supported by woggles (swim noodles) in the water. If this independence does not happen immediately, because your baby still needs physical contact with you, the figures of eight will help you to gain the confidence to handle your baby freely in the water and to take her on and off your back as you start swimming with her.

opening the little harbour

After your baby is stable in the harbour position, with good head control, and is confident with reduced support, holding your arms further apart will stimulate greater movement of your baby's legs and arms in a position that is gradually less upright and more prone in the water. After babies have become used to various movements while being supported in the little harbour, opening it out may trigger various responses.

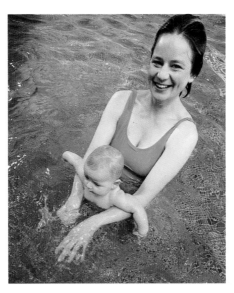

△ **Start from a "little harbour" position with your baby holding herself firmly across your forearms.**

- If your baby is not ready and responds by clinging, return to the little harbour and try again later.
- If your baby launches herself out of your arms with vigorous kicking movements, the next game will be to send her to someone else.
- If your baby is happy being supported between your more widely open arms but does not respond with kicking, then the figures of eight may be the best next step to stimulate leg kicks while continuing to offer support and contact.

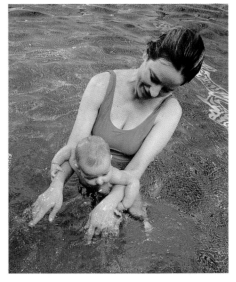

△ **Warn your baby and gradually open your arms wider, letting your baby adjust herself.**

finger hold

Starting from a wide little harbour, lift one bent knee in the water and sit your baby on it. This enables you to remove your arms from under hers for a second and place your index fingers in her hands for her to grab. You are making use of the "palmar grasp" reflex, which makes your baby squeeze your finger when you place it inside her hand. Secure your baby's wrists with your thumbs if necessary. This finger hold is a source of both fun and security. Make sure that your shoulders are relaxed and that you truly let

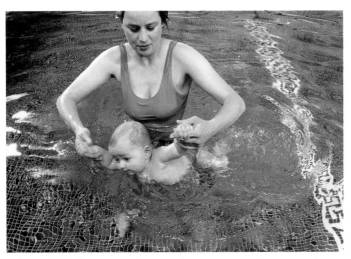

△ **Holding your baby loosely by the index fingers, drag her forwards in the water on her front.**

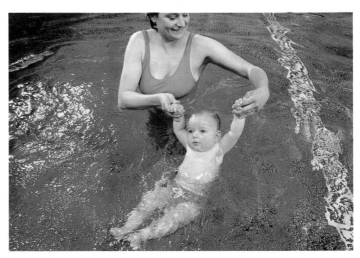

△ **Then, pull her gently backwards and continue the movement back and forth, keeping your baby's body in the water throughout.**

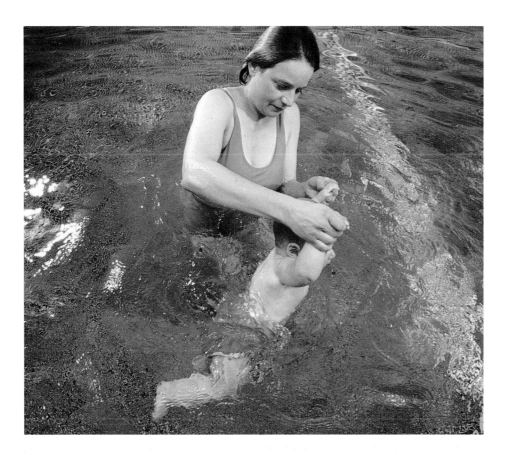

◁ When you are both confident with "finger holding", add a turning movement from the back to the front and again to the back, making figures of eight in the water. Progress from gentle to very energetic movements when your baby is ready.

extended arms, take hold of one of your baby's legs and straighten it. This makes the leg flex or recoil towards her body and then extend again. Straightening one leg after the other encourages your baby to start kicking in the water.

You can also try tickling the soles of your baby's feet, saying the word "kick" as you do it and praising your baby for movement each time. The "kick" word may then become associated with the physical sensation of kicking.

You can also manually help your baby to kick by holding her legs or feet in a semi-supine position in the little harbour and kick them for her, saying "kick, kick" at the same time. After a few times, try saying "kick" to check whether she does or not. You may also place a small ball in front of your baby's feet as a further incentive.

In the figure of eight, you can encourage your baby verbally without manual action by saying "kick" when you notice your baby spontaneously doing a leg kick in the turning movements. Gradually she will associate this action with the word "kick" and learn to recognize it.

▽ In the pre-swimming phase, older babies enjoy kicking while holding on with one finger as they did earlier on.

your baby hold you, keeping the larger part of her body in the water. Try moving her forwards and back so that she experiences the counterflow of the water along her body. With a little practice, your baby alternates between a prone and a supine position.

figure of eight

Once you are confident with this backward and forward swinging movement, you can turn your baby sideways so that she loops from back to front position in a figure of eight. This figure is guided by a wider movement of your outer arm and a smaller movement of your inner arm at each turn. This accustoms your baby to changing positions freely and prepares her for the sensations of swimming. If your baby has lost her amphibian kicking reflex and nothing you do seems to stimulate it, figures of eight may either help to enliven it again or provide an opportunity to establish an association between leg movements and the word "kick" in the transition to voluntary kicking.

from reflex to voluntary leg kicks

First of all, do not worry if kicking is non-existent for several months and your baby just won't do it while others look like

torpedoes in the pool. Some babies just lose their kicking reflex, whatever you do. Be reassured that if you keep taking your baby to the pool, the reflex will appear again as a totally deliberate movement, usually in the second year. When this happens, your toddler will be ready to start swimming. If you wish to encourage your baby to start kicking earlier, there are two things you can do, using both little harbour and figures of eight.

In the little harbour position, a young baby's recoil reflex, which occurs with the amphibian kicking reflex, can be used to stimulate leg kicking. Supporting your baby in a semi-supine position between your

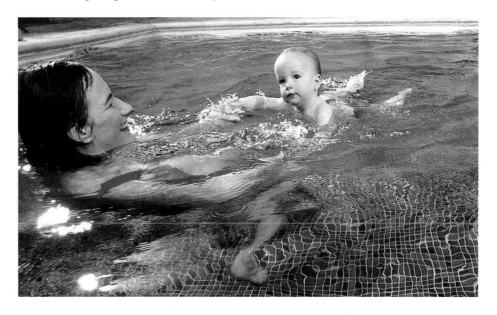

Holding on

After practising the various ways of holding your baby, it is time to teach him to hold on to a bar or a woggle (swim noodle) rather than you. This is a significant step both because of safety and also because your baby is accepting being in the water on his own without physical contact with you. If you remain close and praise achievements, your baby is likely to draw progressively greater strength and confidence even if finding that balance in the water with a support other than your body is not easy at first.

arm support

From an open safety position, encourage your baby to be freer, supported on one of your arms across his chest. The best time to start this is about five to six months, although younger babies may hang happily on to your arm. Moving forward will help your baby to align more easily along the surface rather than hold on to your arm with his body upright in the water. You can continue opening the safety position in wide circular movements, which may also

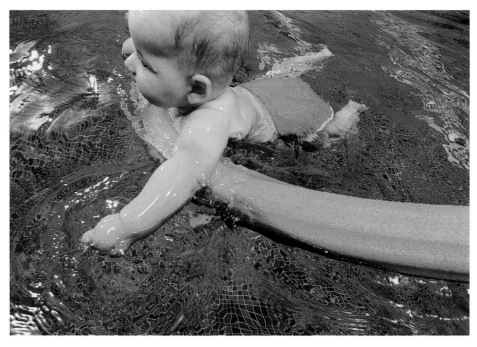

△ **Holding on to foam woggles helps your baby to detach from your body and take control.**

stimulate more kicking. When your baby is confident on your arm, introduce further movement, such as bobbing up and down or zigzagging. These add an element of fun and increase your baby's steadiness.

woggle hold

As soon as your baby is steady in the open safety position, it is a good idea to introduce a foam woggle as a substitute for your arm. Since your baby's balance will be precarious at first, you can hold his arms on the woggle with your thumbs. The sooner you start swimming, with your baby between your arms, your body and the woggle, the more easily your baby will find his balance. When he is able to stretch his body in the water, and even perhaps kick while holding a woggle under his arms, you can place your hands wide apart and gradually remove one hand before, finally, your baby is propelling himself next to you. Another way of using the woggle is to swim on your back and hold your baby's hands while he is supported by a woggle under his arms. Some babies refuse woggles outright. If so, wait two to three weeks before re-introducing them. Your baby may be among those who start swimming without bars or woggles.

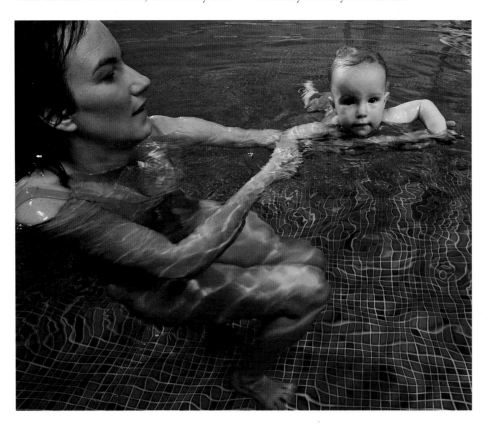

◁ **Giving your baby arm support maintains the close contact that some babies need.**

On the bar

Holding on to the grab bar, if there is one at your chosen pool, is a positive step towards water safety for your baby. From about six months, or whenever he holds on well to your arm, you can start practising placing his hands on the grab bar. If he lets go, catch him calmly and repeat the attempt two or three times. Try again the following week, as it may take a few weeks of trials and practice for your baby to understand what is expected from him. A bar held by two people can be used in pools without a grab bar.

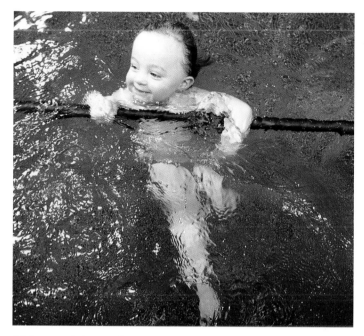

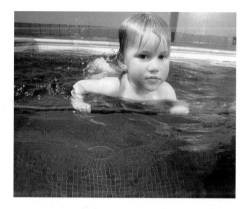

◁ **2** Your baby may respond either by letting go and going under or by tensing up and clinging to the bar in an uncomfortable position. In either case, pick your baby up and place his hands again on the bar in a relaxed way.

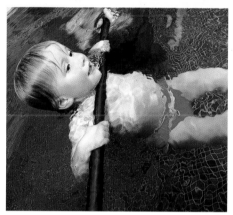

◁ **3** Help your baby by pulling his legs back and kicking them gently. Once your baby holds on, invite him to move his hands along the bar, towards you or to get a toy further along, and to kick and splash, stretching his body in the water.

△**1** Once your baby over six months is happy holding on to your arm, you can try placing his hands on the grab bar or on a bar held by two people in the pool. This may take a few weeks of trials and practice, but your baby will grasp it ultimately. The challenge for your baby is how to avoid disappearing under the bar, because his legs move forward and this makes him tip under.

Woggle support

From early on, you can choose to introduce a water woggle as a substitute support for your arm; this promotes your baby's independence in the water. Before too long, your older baby will find his perfect balance on the woggle. This is one way to unaided swimming; the next step of holding on to the woggle with one arm only is easy once this balance has been gained.

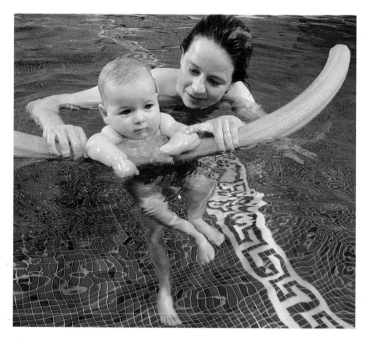

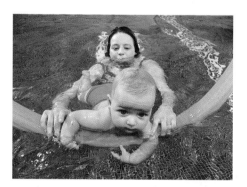

◁ **2** You can then practise all the movements presented on the previous pages or, more interestingly, swim with breaststroke leg movements while holding your baby on the woggle in front of you.

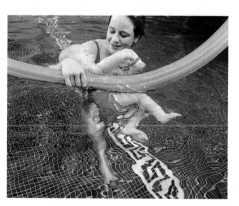

◁ **3** If at any stage your baby goes under because his centre of gravity is not far enough forward, and he tips under the woggle, calmly pick him up, cuddle him and start again.

△**1** Place a woggle across your baby's chest so that his arms rest on it, and stabilize him by placing your hands to either side of his arms or, if he is very young, on his arms.

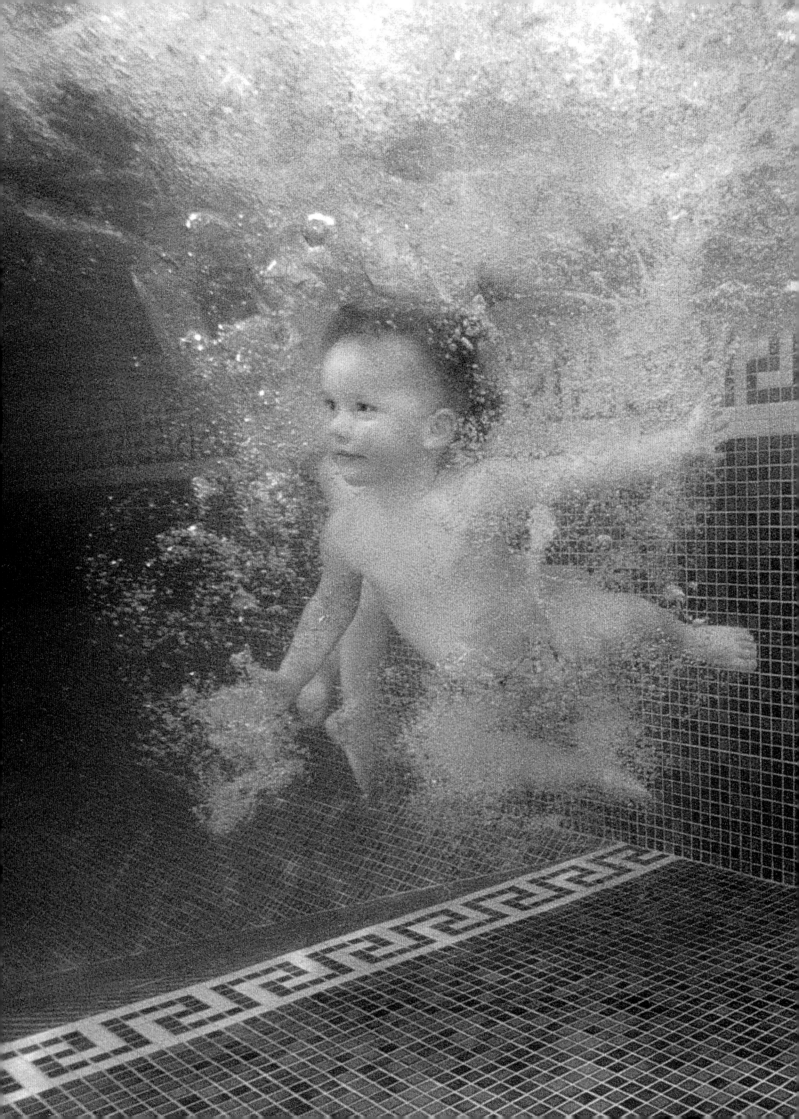

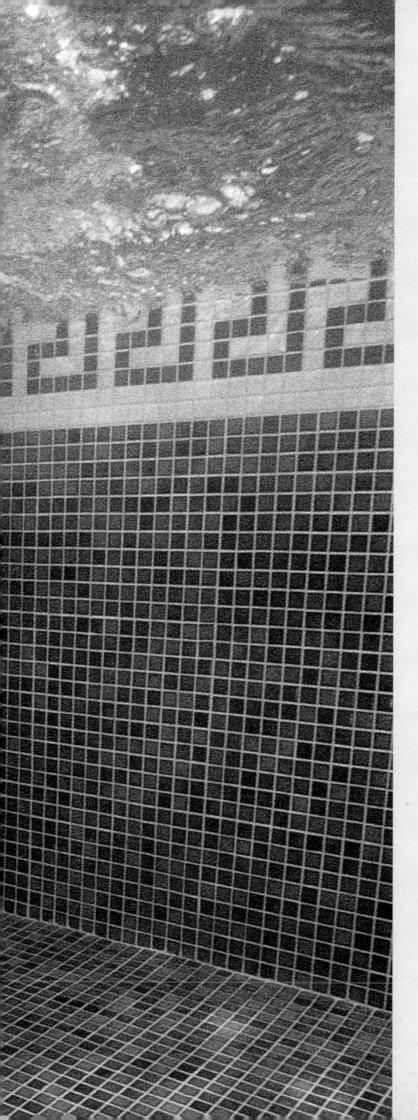

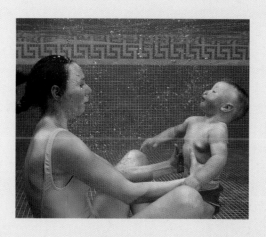

submersion

Up to about six months old, babies have no fear of being underwater. Many babies will move more easily underwater than on the surface. Brief submersions, as described in this chapter, will help to develop your baby's natural ability to swim. Although you may be nervous at first, remember that babies are more ready to enjoy being underwater than adults. Once you realize this, diving with your baby will be a treat.

Relax and watch

To submerge babies safely, parents need to be both relaxed and watchful. There is a mutual process of protecting your vulnerable baby, yet letting her guide you with her new experiences.

their fear, our fear

Can I help my baby to swim without her, or me, needing to go underwater? Take it as a matter of fact that being in the pool with your baby implies that she will go under some time, probably quite soon if it has not already happened. If you are not worried about it, neither will your baby be. As to whether you need to put your face in the water or not, be reassured that this is a matter of choice, although it is preferable that you come to enjoy going under with your child, as babies like the sight of you underwater too.

While submersion is easy with babies under four to five months, it may become more difficult if started later. For older babies, it is best to practice above-water skills for some time and move on to submersion only when you are confident that your baby is happy to put her face in the water and will not be frightened to go

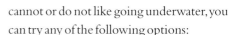

△ The first underwater dip in the pool can be disconcerting for young babies used to submersion in the bath. Eye contact and soft talking can be reassuring.

under. The earlier you start, the easier it is for your baby to be familiar with the underwater world with no fear and with excitement about new experiences. If you start later, building trust and developing skills with the exercises in the previous section are essential for success. If you

cannot or do not like going underwater, you can try any of the following options:

- Be open to experiencing the novelty of submersion with your baby. Forget about difficult past experiences.
- Overcome your resistance by yourself and then practise in the pool with your baby.

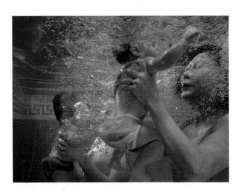

◁ At first, you can hold your baby close to you so that you keep contact with her as you go under together.

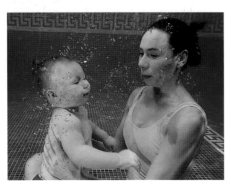

◁ As your baby gets used to going under, you can let her be free for a second or two before bringing her back up to the surface.

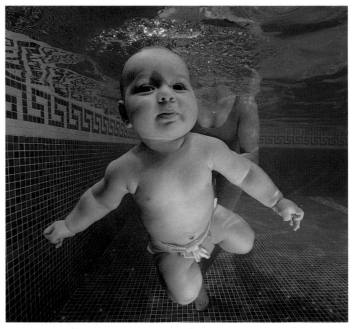

△ Some babies like going underwater more than others – the earlier they start, the easier it seems to be. Never force babies to go underwater if they dislike it.

▷ You may want to go gradually deeper, extending the periods you spend underwater by one second at a time.

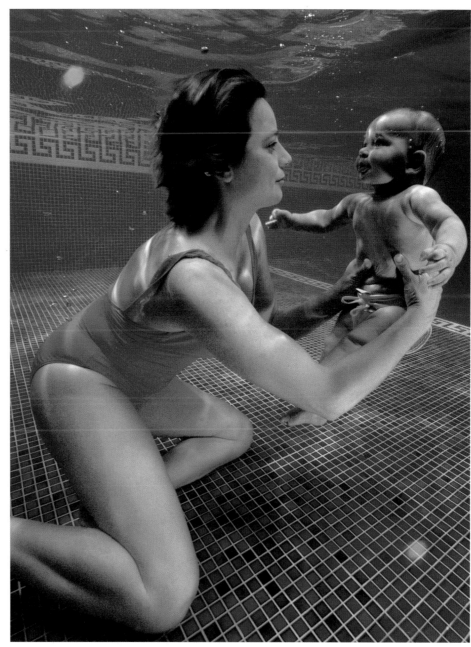

• Admit to your baby that you really do not wish to join in and encourage her to explore the underwater world on her own, praising her for her accomplishments.

Any of these options will help your baby to progress because you are taking a clear stance that will be conveyed to her subconsciously. You will also feel that you have made a choice. Babies seem to be content with any of these options if you are happy with your choice.

being safe

How long can a baby hold her breath? There is no clear answer to this question, as it depends on both age and practice. Do not "water train" your baby by submerging her extensively. Two or three short submersions per session seem sufficient to help your baby to control her breathing underwater and gradually expand her breath-holding capacity week by week. On account of the diving reflex, it is totally safe to submerge babies for two to three seconds at a time, knowing that you have a substantial safety margin. However, do not let your baby be face down or submerged in water for

▷ Babies who need to breathe release bubbles in the water, but if your baby has jumped in, this may not be detectable.

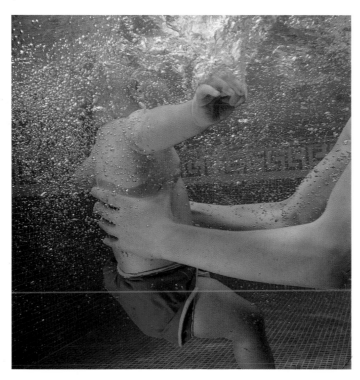

more than a few seconds. If you follow the instructions in this book carefully, submerging will be a safe and happy experience for your baby.

BEING WATCHFUL

This applies to swimming with your baby in general but more particularly to submersion. Whenever your baby goes under, make sure that you are continually checking her wellbeing, albeit in a relaxed rather than anxious manner. By being watchful, you not only ensure that your baby has a pleasant experience, but you also learn to time submersions in relation to your baby's breathing, and you know better when to do it or not, and when to stop.

Ready, steady, go!

By now, your baby's face will have been in the water, doing mini dunks in the bath when he was a newborn or dunking in the front holding position in the pool. It is likely that your baby has already fallen off your arms into the water accidentally during one of the exercises. This may have helped you to realize that going under does not have to be dramatic. Guidelines here are offered to submerge your baby safely and effectively. Hopefully, it will be the beginning of a lifelong enjoyment of diving. Keep in mind that the keys to success are a firm holding, staying calm and moving smoothly and consistently after communicating your intent to your baby.

submerging before five months

Holding your baby firmly under his arms and sending him forward with his face in the water – "dunking" in baby-swimming jargon – is a first step towards submerging very young babies in the pool. This is followed by a duckling dive or submersion together. Submersion can be practised from the first time you take your baby to the pool. At this stage "closing", that is breath control, is automatic, and it is easy for both you and your baby to be relaxed. To a large extent, success is a matter of attitude. Most babies are open to this new experience if it is presented simply. It is good practice to let your baby, even your newborn, know your intent of submerging him. You can do this through eye contact and/or verbally. Young babies also tend to prefer being held closely in their parents' arms. Babies who start submerging from newborn submerge without much change in their faces, although they may come back up with a startled expression after keeping their eyes open underwater.

five months onwards

As your baby will soon have to learn to hold his breath to go underwater when the "gag reflex" has subsided, it is important to find

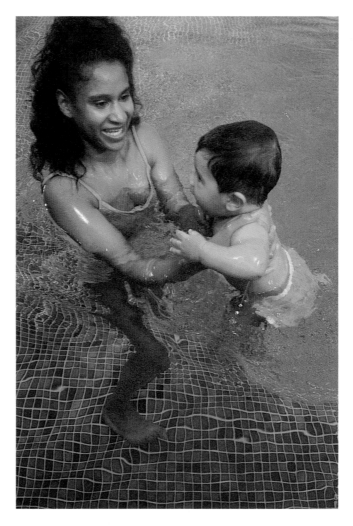

◁ **Signal to your baby that you are about to go underwater by first gaining eye contact, then taking a breath and closing your mouth. Now, without hesitating, lift your baby and submerge him in one smooth movement.**

WARNING
Avoid pressing a young baby's hands when you submerse him – the "Badkin's reflex" makes him automatically open his mouth when you do this, leading to a risk of swallowing water.

ways of prompting him to take a breath and hold it. This will henceforth be called "closing". Babies are good imitators and so you should talk to your baby, get eye contact and then show him how you "close". Remember that babies breathe mostly through their noses throughout their first year. If you cannot take a deep breath through your nose, do so through your mouth. Make sure you close your mouth in any case, because babies who go in the water with their mouths open may swallow some water. To be effective, your action must be immediately followed by submersion so that your baby gets to identify it as a signal. To make it even more effective, you can combine it with a physical movement – for example, a small lift of your baby above the water. Lifting your baby slightly (something

most parents do spontaneously) each time you are ready also signals to him the need to close for imminent submerging. You can also add verbal cues such as "and a one, and a two, and a three, go!"

The sequence then becomes: get eye contact with your baby, take a breath, close your mouth, lift your baby and, without hesitating and in one firm movement, submerge him, preferably with yourself. If your baby tends to swallow water and choke during submersion, it may be helpful to blow in his face to stimulate closing as an automatic response. This is effective but introduces an additional conditioning response that does not seem to be necessary for most babies. Timing is crucial: do not wait for too long between the time when you enlist your baby's readiness to submerge

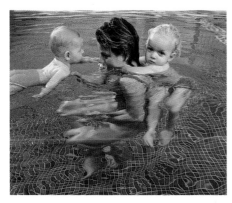

△ **First give a clear signal, facial and verbal, that you are about to submerge.**

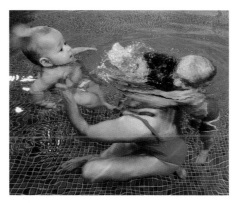

△ **You can also show your baby that you have your mouth closed as you go under.**

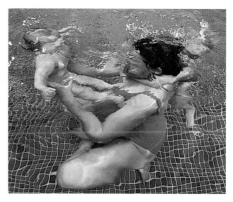

△ **Immediately after your signal, lift your baby slightly and … there you go.**

and the time you do it. This should not be more than a few seconds with a young baby, but may require a little longer with an older baby whom you may need to coax into it. Learn to recognize your baby's own signals of being ready, and practise submerging immediately after he has taken a breath in, timing your signals with his breathing. Do not hesitate, as this will confuse your baby. Once you have made your "ready" signal, you have communicated that going underwater is imminent and you have to follow suit. Two or three times per session are enough at the beginning.

steady and firm

Whatever your baby's age, a steady, calm, firm hold will add to the experience of submerging and increase your baby's confidence. Holding your baby firmly may give him the first cue of all that precedes submersion. Make a continuous movement from start to finish, without any sudden interruption, and always end with a hug or kiss. If it helps, you can count to three before

you start the movement back out rather than feeling you must bring your baby back up instantly. Do not jerk your baby out of the water with a sudden, anxious movement, as this may alarm him.

go deep enough

Many parents do not submerge their babies deep enough at first. A shallow submersion in which your baby's head is not underwater can be confusing and uncomfortable for your baby. From the start, make sure that your baby's whole head is submerged.

using rhythm

Repetitive movement seems to be very conducive to easy submerging. Small jumps, without splashing, holding your baby closely while going up and down with a rapid tempo are very popular. When your baby is used to the rhythmical movement, look at him to get his attention and submerge him, then, as you come back up, hug him and continue jumping. When several parents and babies do this in a circle,

jumping in a clockwise motion, a collective effect is added and babies rarely cry. Always have a cuddle at the end and move to a quiet activity afterwards.

well done!

Greet and praise your baby on the way out of the water. If he is crying for any reason, resist holding him too tightly as if he had just been rescued. If you were apprehensive and you have to slow down your own heart beat, now is the time to relax.

At first, babies often emerge with a disorientated look from this intense adjustment to a range of new sensations. As you greet them cheerfully, they soon get used to the transition between being above and beneath the surface of the water.

If your baby cries on two successive submersions, comfort him gently, allow him to settle down and do not attempt submersion again until the following session. You may have to take particular care to ensure that an older baby is happy to try again next time.

WATER INTOXICATION

Extremely high levels of water in the body can cause water intoxication (hyponatremia, also known as "dry drowning"). It can affect babies and small children if they swallow excessive amounts of water in swimming pools. The symptoms, which appear later on at home, are sickness and lethargy. Do not be alarmed, as this potentially dangerous condition is rare. Your baby will not be at risk if you follow these instructions for submerging:

• Always make sure your baby is happy between submersions.
• Do not use repeated, frequent submersions in one session.
• Stop submerging if your baby is distressed.
• Show your baby how to "blow out" water early on.

▷ **The two keys to successful submersion are to be prompt and steady, and to go deep enough. A tentative, shallow submersion is less comfortable for your baby. Count one, two, three, then come back up slowly.**

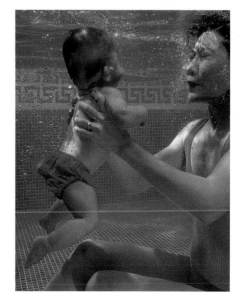

Going underwater

Being firm and bold from the very first time you submerge your baby enables her to be familiar with the water environment with ease and comfort. As you become familiar with submerging, you can see your baby looking at you underwater. You can both explore this different environment, which offers distinct sensations. A few babies resist submersion until they start swimming in their second or third year; do not force your baby, as respecting her resistance may be more fruitful in the long term.

going deeper

As you both gain confidence, you can go deeper and extend the time you spend underwater. You can also let your baby go under and come up by herself. Take your time to be comfortable and proceed gradually but, at the same time, try and remain very relaxed while being watchful. In a shallow pool, sitting at the bottom of the

pool is a good way to make sure you go deeper. Your baby enjoys looking around and seeing you if you are underwater too. Older babies may also enjoy going to visit underwater lights on the pool walls or recognizing colourful toys that you may submerge for them.

breath control

Many adults do not like going underwater because of early unhappy experiences with breathing. Submersion is the simplest form of breath control, the most effective, easiest way of increasing your baby's breath-holding capacity without any effort in the transition from reflexive to automatic holding of the breath. It contributes to making later swimming a positive experience.

Older babies soon learn to control their breathing as the amount of time they spend underwater is gradually extended. Neither babies nor adults use the maximum capacity

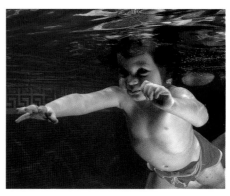

△ **Babies approaching their first birthday enjoy propelling themselves towards the surface.**

of their lungs, so six or seven seconds will not harm a baby over six months, but will allow her to use more of her lung capacity.

Do not, however, try to increase your baby's breath-holding capacity by increasing the amount of time your baby is held underwater. Instead, gradually take a little longer to be with your baby underwater so that this becomes familiar. Knowing when to stop is important with submersion. Some babies enjoy going under so much that they are keen to do it again and again, and do not want to stop. Watch for the first signs that your baby may have had enough, and quit before overtiredness occurs.

When does my baby need to take a breath and what if she takes a breath underwater?
Many babies breathe at irregular intervals in and out of the water. Try and recognize the signs that she will soon need a breath – these are blowing bubbles and frantic movements that may resemble the early amphibian kicking reflex. Bring your baby up immediately. With deeper submersions, if you see bubbles coming out of your baby's mouth and nose, it is time to come up to the surface. Bubbles indicate that your baby is exhaling and that she will soon need to take another breath. However, parents rarely need to rely on these signs unless they keep their babies under for more than a few seconds, which is not advisable. Take your time before adding on each second.

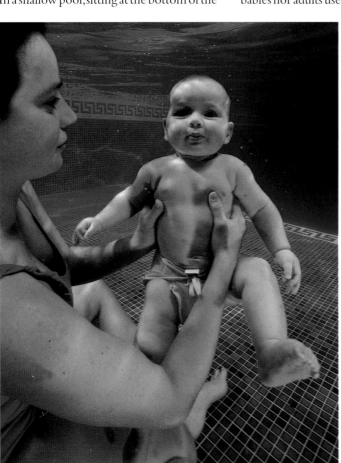

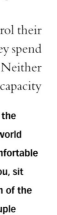

◁ **As visiting the underwater world becomes comfortable for both of you, sit at the bottom of the pool for a couple of seconds.**

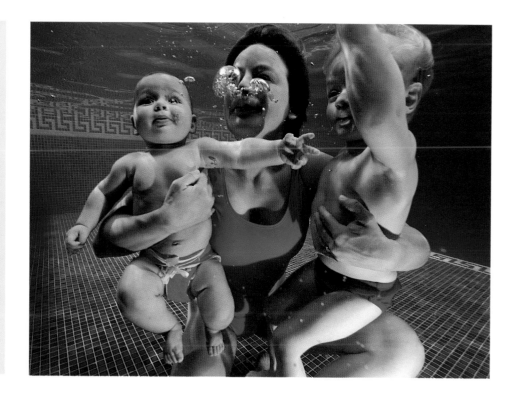

HEALTH CONCERNS

If your older baby has been diagnosed with asthma, check with your doctor that it is all right to take your baby swimming. Submersion can help to reduce the symptoms of asthma in small children who have already been diagnosed as asthmatic. Breath control in submersion may be a positive experience for babies growing up in a family with a history of asthma. Submersion does not seem to aggravate or increase the occurrence of lung or bronchial problems or any tendency to ear infections. Babies should avoid the pool when they have infections until they have fully recovered.

My baby keeps swallowing water every time we go under. What should I do?

Except on rare occasions when babies have blocked nostrils, they breathe through their noses and they do not take in water even if their mouths are open. The first thing is to check their nasal passages. If your baby chokes when going underwater, you can try and encourage her to "close" on an inhalation, signalling submersion precisely at this time. With practice, you can listen to your baby's chest and produce this signal as you hear her take a breath, so that submersion coincides with the end of her in-breath. If your baby continues to choke, it may be helpful to seek medical advice, as there may be a physiological reason that interferes with your baby's ability to hold her breath underwater.

Some babies take in water through their mouths more easily than others and swallow it when they go under. If you notice that your baby keeps swallowing water, systematically show your baby how

CHEERS!

If your baby chokes and spits out water, do not make an alarmed, distressed expression, which may worry her. It is a healthy process, which you should acknowledge as such, and congratulate with a sense of humour.

you close your mouth before submersion and train her to blow out in the water. Until your baby has learnt not to swallow water, you should limit the time and number of submersions in order to avoid any risk of water intoxication.

- Show your baby how close your mouth in a theatrical, fun way.
- Show your baby how to blow in the water at each session as well as at home in the bath. Buy a bubble blowing kit.
- Go a little deeper each session, as babies often learn to close their mouths more easily during deeper submersions.
- If you find that your baby has trouble closing during alternate horizontal and vertical submersions, perhaps because she objects to water going up her nose, move on directly to dives.

surfacing

Submersion is an important water-safety skill that gives older babies control of their breathing underwater in a relaxed way and trains them to surface without panic. Once this is acquired and combined with the skill of holding on, a small child has a much better chance of survival should she accidentally fall in the water. After only a few submersions, some babies start associating going underwater with movement towards the surface. This may be the way that an older baby, over eight months, discovers swimming.

△ **Babies like to go under together – you can make it a family trip.**

Once your baby is confident and happy with submersion, from sitting at the bottom of the pool with your baby, allow her to surface. Your baby may rise quickly; be ready to catch her as soon as she surfaces, pick her up gently as she slows down, just under the surface, and praise her. After your older baby can propel herself to the surface, be watchful in case you need to help her, but allow her to find her way without snatching her ahead of time.

You can develop your baby-surfacing skills by combining submersion with jumps from four months and with throws from six months onwards.

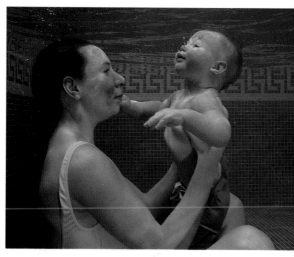

△ **From six months onwards, start releasing your baby gradually to encourage surfacing.**

Duckling dives

Baby dives propel your baby underwater head first. The benefits are numerous and long-lasting. Babies learn to put their heads in the water at the most efficient angle for swimming, which gives them a foundation for aligning their body correctly without straining their necks, and promotes a most efficient and relaxed swimming style. Many babies learn swimming from the dives, moving gradually closer and closer to the surface until they are strong enough to raise their faces for breathing. Dives use a horizontal force, propelling your baby

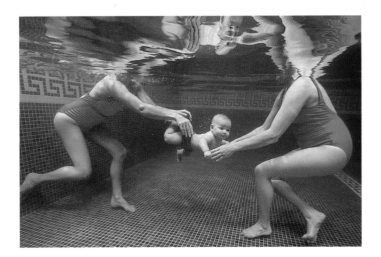

◁ **In the first duckling dives, babies move safely from the arms of one adult to another, being gently caught just after being launched.**

First dives

Your baby is now ready to take his first plunge into the underwater world.

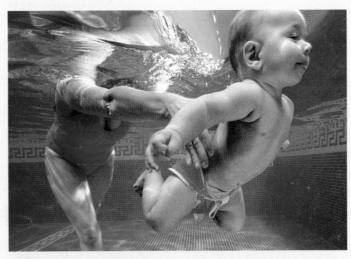

△ **Make sure that your baby's head is completely submerged.**

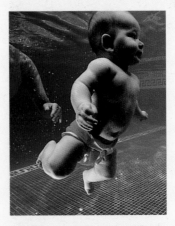

△ **Follow your baby's orientation while he is underwater.**

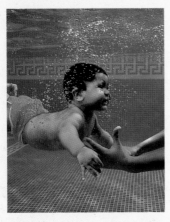

△ **An energetic propelling creates a better dive for your baby.**

1 Stand about 1–2m/3–6ft apart, facing the person who will receive your baby. Hold your baby at your side and facing away from you. Agree with the other adult about timing – for example, counting "one, two, three" during the dive.

2 Holding your baby under his arms, tilt him slightly downward to prepare him for a dive. Turn him briefly towards you to signal "closure" and push him down gently but firmly towards your partner underwater, rather deeper than just under the surface.

3 At first, your baby moves rapidly between your hands and the welcoming hands of your partner. Gradually increase this space, propelling your baby more strongly and watching his movement. If your baby happens to flip over underwater and finds himself face up or sideways, pick him up gently and calmly.

4 Try and observe your baby's movements in the water:
- Is he moving at all?
- Does he tend to roll over on his back?
- Does he tend to surface during the dive?
- Does he emerge happy?

Always greet your baby and praise him with your warmest tone of voice when he emerges. If your baby choked, make sure you pay close attention to his breathing next time, and submerge him just after he has taken a breath.

5 If you are on your own, hold your baby at arms' length facing you. Signal submersion, lift and propel your baby towards you, face down, underwater. Step back if needed. Pick him up gently, praise and cuddle him. As your confidence grows, step back further.

6 With older babies, you can push them more, which is good practice for directing themselves to the edge. You can hold a toy just under the surface for your baby to reach.

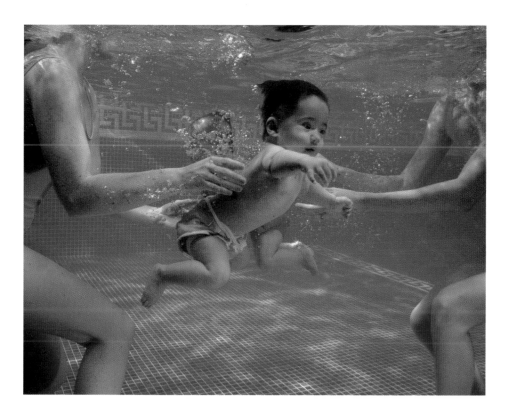

remember that they are not necessarily conducive to swimming unaided and can even detract from early swimming.

How far apart should parents or friends be?

This depends on your baby's age, breathing capacity and motor development. With a young baby under five months, frantic arm and leg reflex movement indicates that your baby needs to breathe and must be picked up; the distance between you and your baby's receiver is probably too great. With an older baby, watch the development of deliberate "pulling" arm movements to reach out towards you or the other person. It is then time to increase the gap to allow your baby full scope for expanding his arm movements, and your baby is on the way to unaided swimming. The beginning of dog paddling in baby dives often starts true co-ordinated swimming. Holding a toy about 30cm/12in underwater as a target for your older baby and giving it to him to surface with is a first step towards the future enjoyment of retrieving objects underwater.

▽ Welcoming your baby from beneath the surface makes a duckling dive a joint adventure.

forward; this anticipates the feeling of swimming later on. Dives initiate babies to the joy of diving and motivate them to balance their bodies in the water and find their orientation as soon as they gain control of their leg movements later in their first year.

swapping babies

If you are in the pool with a friend and her baby, you can swap babies in the dives. Facing each other, send your baby to your friend on your right or left, and agree that she will send her baby to you on the same side to avoid clashes. The babies then come back to their respective parents. Babies can also be passed in dives from parent to parent in a small circle. Stop the game if a baby cries and needs repatriating for a cuddle.

How deep beneath the water should I push my baby?

It is easier to practise with deeper dives at first so that your baby is completely submerged. Later, when your baby starts "swimming" towards a target, encourage shallow dives to facilitate later surfacing. It is fine to continue deep dives for fun, but

DOES YOUR BABY KEEP HIS EYES OPEN UNDERWATER?

Encourage your older baby to reach for you or a toy, or the grab bar, as a step towards pulling up for something to hold on to while taking a breath. Check the water balance by opening your eyes too. If your eyes get sore, perhaps it will soon be time to buy your baby his first pair of goggles. Some babies do not like opening their eyes underwater. Check if they do so at home in the bath to find out if this is their preference or a sensitivity to the pool water. Overall, it is better for your baby to develop an early habit of keeping his eyes open underwater.

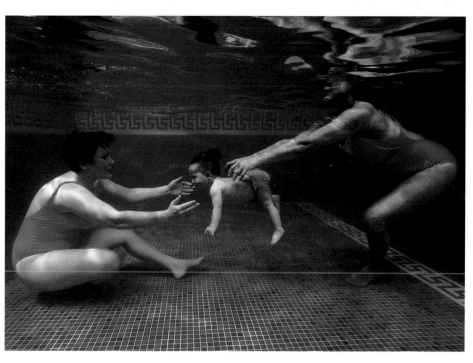

Front dives

If you are confident underwater and your baby has got used to duckling dives, you can move on to front dives, in which you submerge together with your baby, holding her in front of you and taking a dive that takes you under and back up to the surface again. Your dive can be shorter or longer according to what you and your baby are ready for at the time. This is a way to get your baby used to deeper submersions in which she is propelled forward with greater force than in the duckling dives. Front dives are best done with babies over five months who start enjoying movement and the discovery of the world around them.

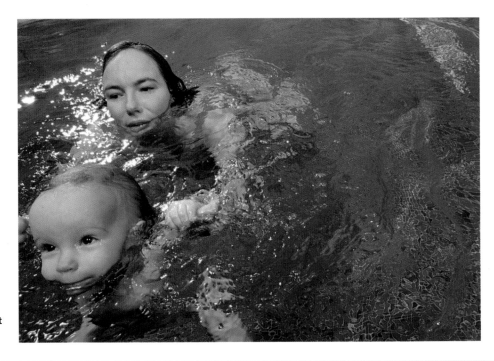

▷ **Swimming across the pool with your baby in front of you combines strong movement and short dives.**

Short front dive
You and your baby can both enjoy the thrill of gliding through the water as you practise front dives.

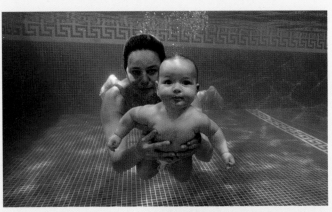

◁ **Take a firm launch, pushing against the pool wall with your feet well under the surface.**

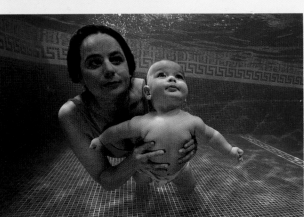

▷ **As you both come up at the end of your dive and surface, swim if you can hold your baby above water.**

1 Standing in the pool, hold your baby under her arms facing outwards. Turn her to have eye contact for a moment and signal closure, taking a deep breath and closing your mouth.

2 Immediately, with your baby facing forward again, go under, holding her in front of you. In a pool where the water reaches your chest, you may also take a little jump to take a head-first dive.

3 If you find this difficult, submerge with your baby and push with your feet on the pool floor to finish your dive and move back up. With practice, you can obtain a smooth movement into the underwater world and out again. This often makes your baby kick back as you surface, and prepares her to surface by herself from dives and jumps. If your baby takes off in a flurry of kicking movements as you both surface, why not swim with her as long as you can until you both go under again.

▷ **For a more energetic dive, swim underwater with your baby, and surface together after a few strokes. Strong swimmers need to be responsive to their babies' enjoyment of dives at any time, and never use force.**

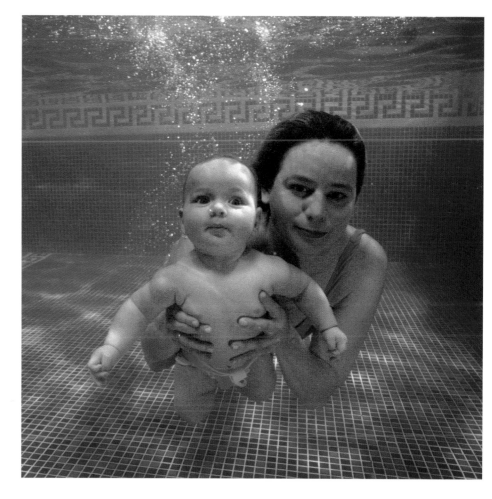

long front dive

In this dive, you extend the time that you and your baby spend underwater and you cover a greater distance as you swim with your legs while holding your baby in front of you. You need to be a confident swimmer and diver. This can be a quite dynamic adventure in which you take your baby below the surface with you to explore the pool floor or lighting, or simply to enjoy movement underwater together. Some babies do not seem to get tired from front dives, but it is prudent not to do more than two or three in one session.

You can either hold your baby in front of you with two hands or under one arm on the side, which liberates your other arm. Holding your baby with one arm makes it easier to take a deeper front dive, as you can use your free arm to lead your dive.

dives from floats

With older babies, front dives can be encouraged from large floats or from inflatable toys. Even before babies are able to sit up, you can hold them on the edge of a float and allow them to drop gently into the water head first. When babies are able to sit up by themselves, small movements of the float will make them fall forward and take a dive. If you pick your baby up slowly and calmly, cheering and welcoming her, this becomes a favourite game. In *Birthlight* classes, it has proved to be the easiest way to cajole older babies and toddlers into taking their first dives without fear, particularly when they do not like jumping or have become bored with jumping from the wall. Front dives from floats are a very enjoyable way of increasing the distance, step by step, between you and your baby as she starts propelling herself in the water towards you from the dive. Taking dives from floats also offers opportunities for social games, since several babies can sit together and dive in turn whenever the movements of the float make them drop in. If your baby starts to show any signs of feeling insecure and of not enjoying the rough and tumble of these diving games, you should stop them for a while, and try once again a couple of months later.

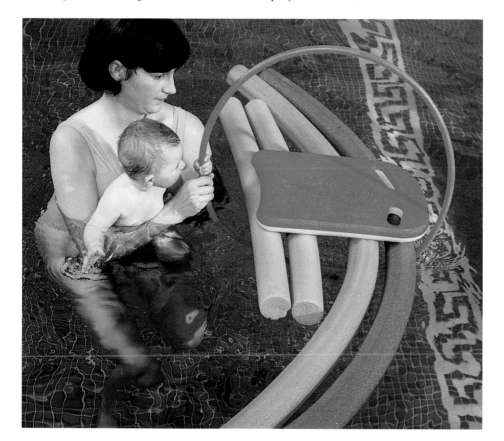

◁ **Most babies will enjoy the sensation of falling gently from the edge of a float, as they take their first moves towards diving.**

Jumping from the wall

From a sitting position on the edge of the pool, jumping is another approach to submersion that suits some babies best, particularly older ones who require a greater consolidation of trust before they can enjoy going under. Jumping can be practised from the start with young babies who can be held on the edge of the pool long before they can sit. Jumping stimulates the process of coming up to the surface and it can be practised either as a separate skill or, even better, linked with swimming across the pool taking a front ride with you.

Encouraging your baby to let himself fall from the edge of the pool into the water, first held in your arms and then by himself into your arms, until later he jumps in with tremendous splashes, is a path of trust that builds confidence in both you and your baby. Always praise the performance of your baby, even on off days, and ackowledge any fear of jumping without making an issue of it, reaffirming your unconditional love.

come on!

Except for very small babies, who should be held all the time, place your baby right on the edge of the pool and let him fall in, catching him just as he reaches the water. The slightest wriggle forward allows your baby to fall into the pool, which may

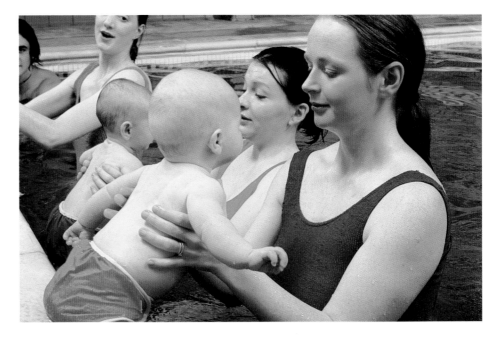

become a great game. Be careful with grab bars or gullies, and if either is prominent, it is better to hold him while he falls or jumps. Welcome your baby into your arms with smiling praise, gradually letting him dip more into the water until he no longer minds jumping into the water unaided and then being picked up by you as he surfaces.

come swimming

Whether you have to help your baby to jump in or he has taken the leap by himself, you can take off swimming on your back

△ **Invite your baby to jump in, keeping eye contact and talking to build up trust in this daring leap forward.**

just after you welcome him into the pool. This gives him a pleasant feeling of jumping to swim with you. Then, you can cross the pool and when you arrive at the other side, sit him on the edge, ready to start a new crossing. Most babies enjoy this game a lot, and this motivates them to be more and more relaxed in their approach to jumping towards you.

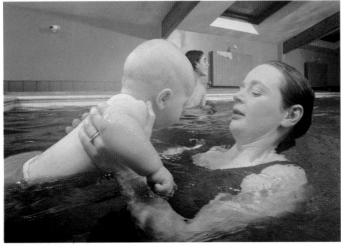

△ **As soon as your baby jumps in, take off on your back, holding him loosely on top of you to begin with and gradually letting go.**

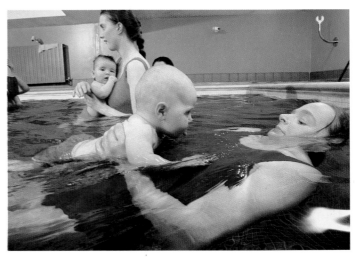

△ **With practice, you will soon become able to swim across the pool. Repeat jumping and taking off from the other side of the pool.**

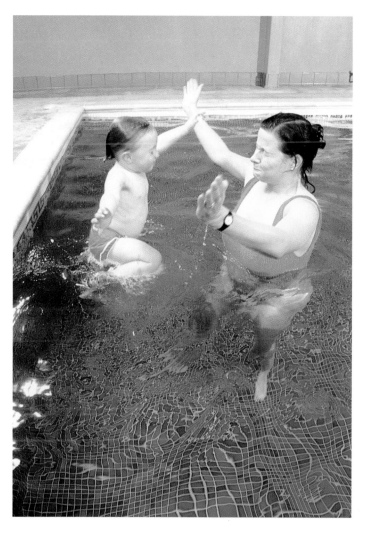

Some older babies need coaxing with a finger or a game of hand clapping. At the beginning, babies can be held or caught just above the surface of the water rather than submerged, but progressively they can be allowed to go under before being picked up. Eventually, allow your baby to go right under and surface alone. Jumping is an enjoyable game in which going underwater is part of throwing oneself to disappear and then reappear to find Mother or Father there. Vertical submersions prepare babies to be active and involved in jumps early on.

With advanced babies who have started propelling themselves in the duckling dives, parents can step back a little and encourage their babies to swim towards them after jumping in. Babies may start swimming after jumping by themselves and striving to reach parents in the water.

◁ **From one finger hold to no finger at all, older babies love throwing themselves into the water. Cheer them as they surface!**

▽ **When babies take tremendous splashing jumps, they can be encouraged to propel themselves towards you as they surface.**

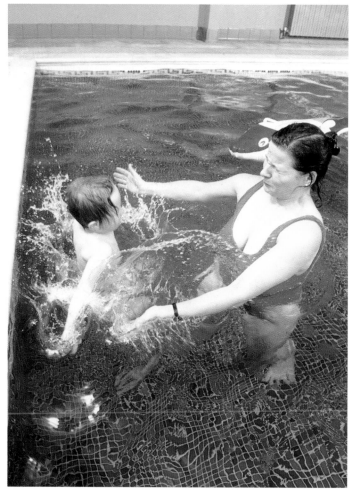

SAFETY PRECAUTIONS

- Note the height of the edge, and any prominent bar or gully.
- When babies are able to stand alone, you can hold their hand while standing in the pool and help them to jump well clear of the edge.
- If your baby wishes to jump from a standing position, place a hand behind his lower back to ensure his balance before he jumps. Give him a hand or finger to hold to make sure that he jumps well clear of the pool wall or grab bar.
- Jumping can become such a thrill for some babies that they throw themselves off the side without watching if a parent is there to welcome them. At this stage it is important to develop safety skills such as holding on to the edge or bar, back floats and swimming to the side. It may be necessary to hold such babies and direct them systematically to the side each time they jump in, particularly if they are also reluctant to hold on to your body while you swim. You can also aim at training your baby to wait for a particular signal to jump to an adult in the water. Taking prompt action is preferable to scaring your baby with cries of alarm as he goes near the pool.
- Toddlers may become strong enough to climb out of the pool by themselves and want to jump in again. From the first instance, it is important to make a decision about encouraging or discouraging this practice. Some pools do not allow standing jumps.

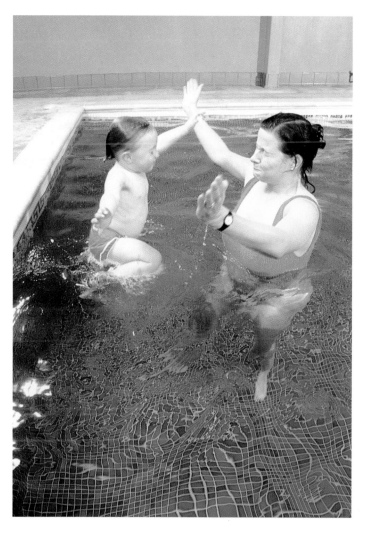

Baby throws

Throwing your older baby up in the air and gradually letting her submerge from an increasing height, provided she enjoys it as many babies do, is a way to increase your baby's confidence with submersion and surfacing in a playful, active way. It familiarizes your baby with being above and below the water surface intermittently, holding her breath automatically to go under, taking a breath when surfacing. She learns to use her legs and arms to surface, which is made easier as the high throw increases her buoyancy. High throws also teach your baby not to be afraid of entering the water from a height of up to 1m/3ft and going deep underwater before moving up to surface. They stimulate stronger leg kicks, extend babies' capacity to hold their breath

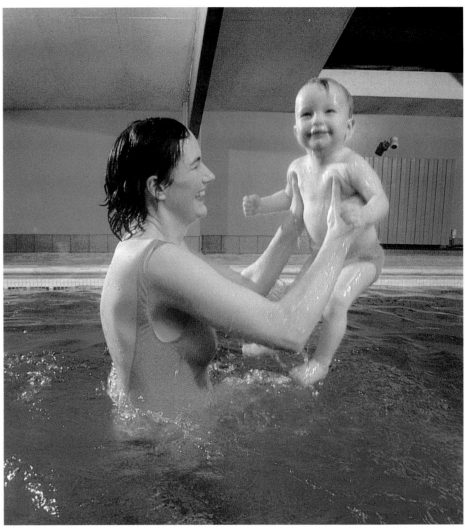

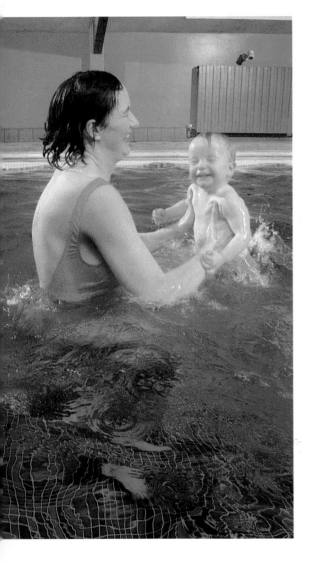

underwater and accustom them to surface without any fear. At the beginning, it is better for you to go under as well in order to check your baby's movement and monitor her surfacing. With practice, you can welcome her when she surfaces, picking her up immediately and giving her a cuddle and the usual praise. Later, when your baby has acquired enough strength to pull herself up towards you, help her to do so by giving her just as much support as she may need, from two hands to a little finger. After your baby has taken a breath, you can also step back and drag her for a short swim, or jump again.

◁ **Prepare your baby for a high throw with several small bouncing movements, which help her to anticipate your action.**

△ **To reassure your baby, lift her gently and drop her slowly and calmly back into the water.**

the advantages

Baby throws are a dynamic way to get cautious babies and fearful older babies to enjoy submerging. You can make them secure by holding your baby all the way at first and only "throw" her up and let her jump in from above when she is completely happy about the movement and shows every sign of enjoying it.

High throws can be very enjoyable for both you and your baby, but you must be careful not to overdo them, as in the middle of having fun it is easy to overlook the amount of time spent underwater and your baby may get more tired than you think.

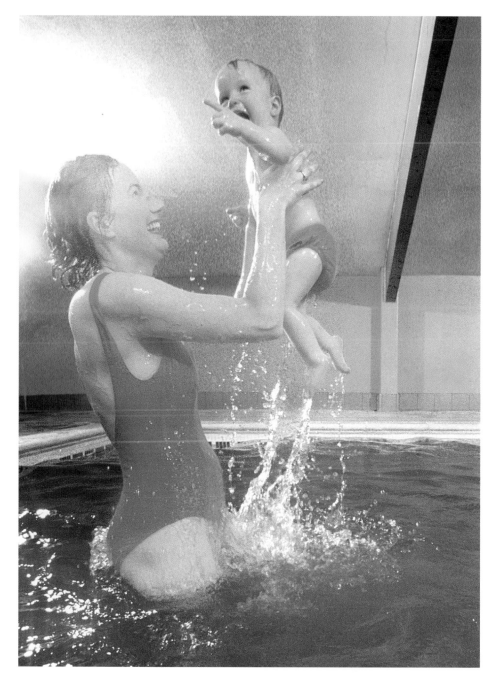

◁ **When your baby is confident, actively throw her up in the air. At first, catch her in your arms before dipping her again. Later on, when she is ready, let her go in from the full height.**

▽ **Watch your baby surface from a throw, and wait until she emerges before picking her up.**

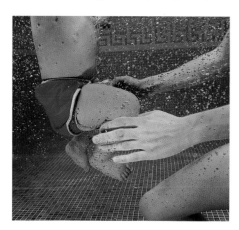

times, they help to build up the strength she needs to start swimming and develop both her skills and her confidence through play. This can be a special opportunity to start your own water games, which you can develop together week by week during your visits to the pool.

For older babies and toddlers, water games add incentives for going to the pool at times when progress appears to be slow in the pre-swimming phase. Games strengthen the love bond between you and your baby, and remind you that enjoying your time at the pool together comes before performance.

water games

Older babies who do not mind submerging can have great fun with water toys. After the three forms of submersion have been practised to the point where your baby or toddler is totally relaxed with "falling in", games with surf boards and inflatables can make your visit to the pool more lively, and create a diversion in your routine practice. They help your baby to regain her balance whichever way she goes under, even if she finds herself in awkward positions under the inflatables. While you need to supervise such games very closely and be ready to pick up your baby at all

▷ **Develop your child's strength and confidence by introducing water games.**

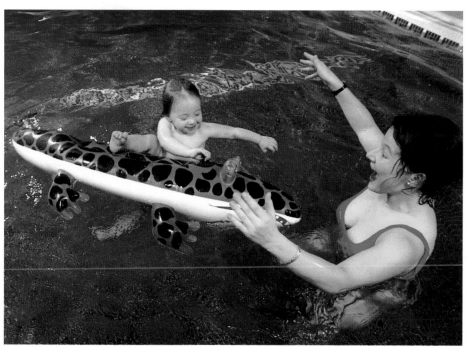

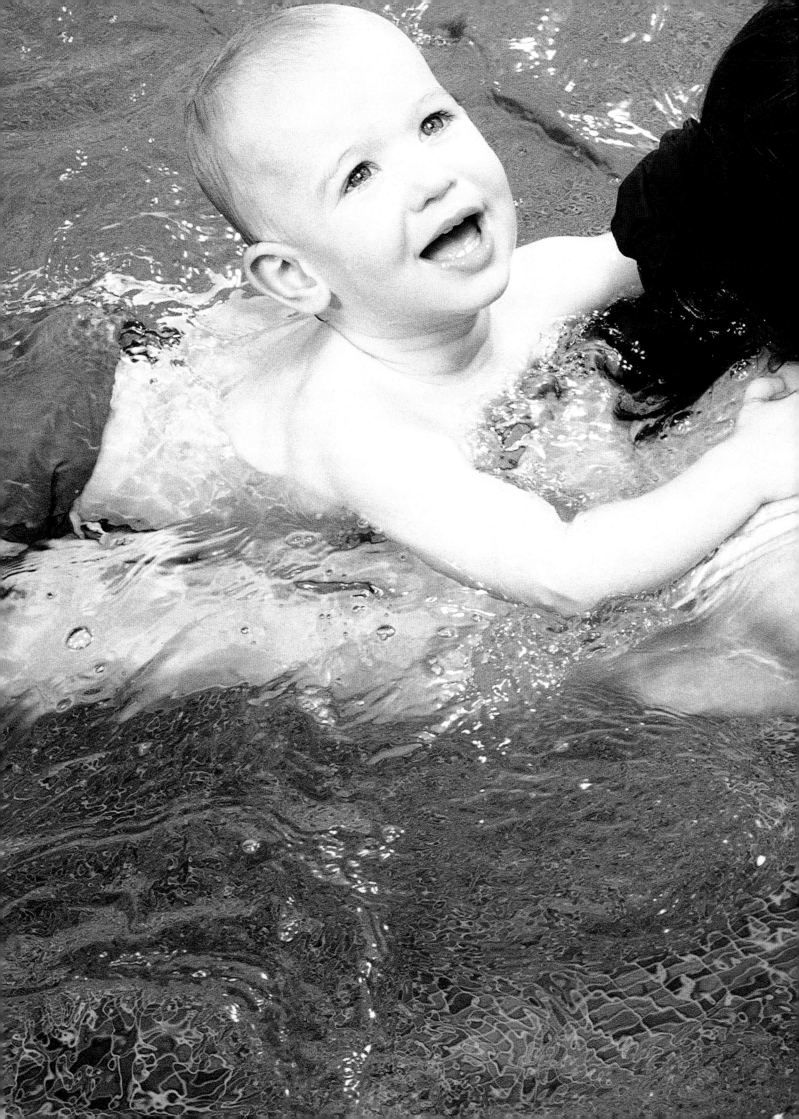

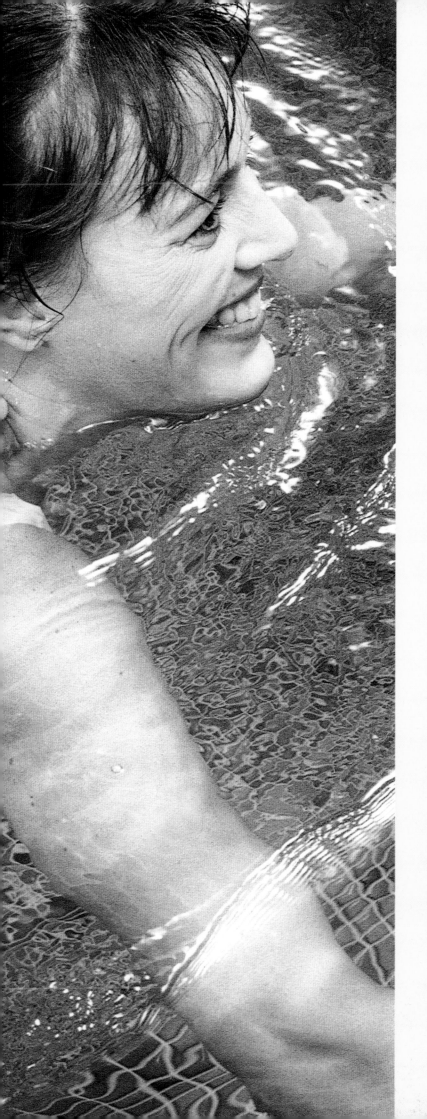

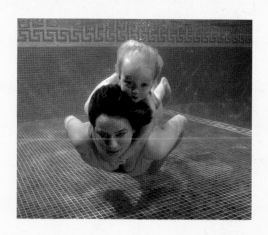

swimming
with
babies

For centuries, Amazonian parents have carried their babies on their backs when swimming in rivers or lakes. This is often the baby's first experience of water. There is no reason why we should not do this too. After a little practice, swimming with your baby, first on your front, then on your back, will be easy and fun – an intimate adventure for both of you to share, whether travelling a tiny distance or the entire length of the pool.

Supported and free front rides

From a back float you can take off for a "front ride" while holding your baby on your chest. At first, while you are gaining confidence and getting used to having your baby on your body, a support may be helpful – you can either use a foam board (kickboard), which you place on your front for your baby to rest on, either on his back or on his front, or one or two water woggles (swim noodles) under your arms to increase your buoyancy. Make sure you place your baby higher rather than lower on your chest in front rides, as babies have a tendency to slip down as you swim.

with a board under your back

Firstly, get comfortable with the feeling of having your baby on your body during a back float. Have a board under your lower back to give you support if needed. At first, getting into a back swimming position with a young baby may be daunting. If you are not very confident in water, ask someone to place the baby on your body once you are in a comfortable position and to watch you while you take off. Boards, however, need to be positioned carefully under your lower back to stay in place and give you freedom of movement. Unless your board is in the position that is right for

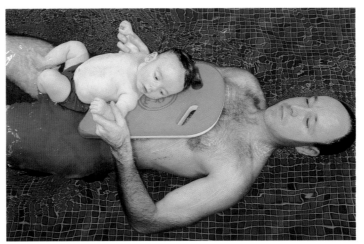

your back, it may slip out of place, which can result in an unexpected submersion. If this happens, hold on to your baby and regain your footing calmly. Once you have adjusted your board, this can be a relaxing way to start swimming with a baby resting on your body.

with a board over your chest

If having a board under your back does not suit you, you can place your baby on the board on top of you in order to have more buoyancy. You may feel more steady this way. Even though your baby is not in direct contact with your body, you can hold his body or just his hands. You can also sprinkle water gently on his tummy as you swim

along. It is important that the air temperature is high enough for comfort if you swim in this way with a young baby.

with water woggles

Another way of supporting yourself on your back to give your baby a front ride is to place one or more water woggles under your arms. Try several positions for your baby on your chest, on his front and on his back. The support of the woggles enables you to lessen your hold on your baby over time, leaving him free to find his own balance. Parents can make good use of front rides with their babies to tone their abdominal muscles with back crawl leg kicks up and down the pool.

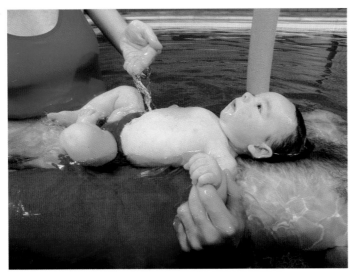

△ A board or woggle positioned under your lower back allows your baby to rest directly on your chest and abdomen.

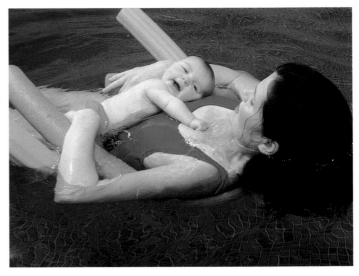

△ Water woggles offer more buoyancy still, and are ideal for parents who are not water-confident.

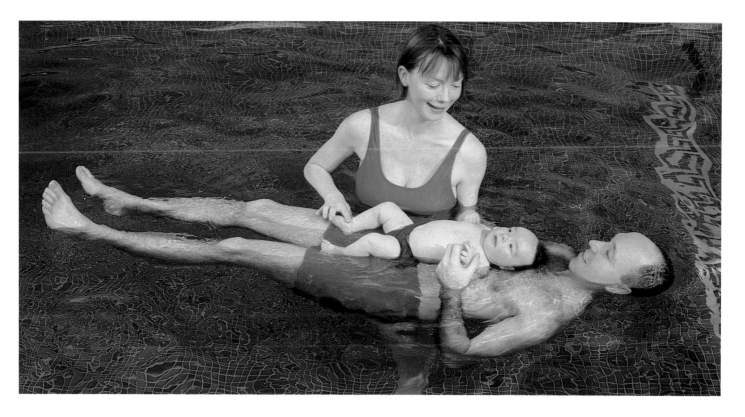

free front rides

If you are water-confident, swimming with your baby on your front is largely a matter of allowing your body to relax with him rather than tensing up. The more you relax, the better you float and the more enjoyable swimming with your baby gets. Gradually you come to realize that your baby does not need to be held and that you can swim freely together. Front rides allow both closeness and self-reliance, as your baby takes charge of himself, yet is in close contact with you. Swimming around the pool soon evolves from a risky ride to an exciting adventure, and finally becoming a special treat for the older baby.

learning to let go

As you take off on your back, hold your baby on either side of his rib cage. Putting his chest or back on your breastbone usually ensures a steady position. Slowly remove your hands, keeping them close at first and then using them to paddle along. Try not to tense up and make a point of relaxing, which your baby will enjoy. If your baby slips down on to your abdomen, bring your arms up to hold him and lift him back on to your chest.

free ride

Once your baby is used to your swimming movement, little can phase him in front rides. He will become more and more at

△ Parents can help each other to install their baby in a relaxed floating position.

ease, often smiling to other people in the pool and sometimes even taking off by himself to catch a ball that may be floating by. Then you know the time has come to use the front rides mainly for comfort and as an intimate treat while your focus becomes your baby's transition to swimming. Front rides also offer a different challenge to babies over five months. If you start front rides with a baby who dislikes being on his back, place him prone on your front, as high on your chest as possible, letting him hold on to you.

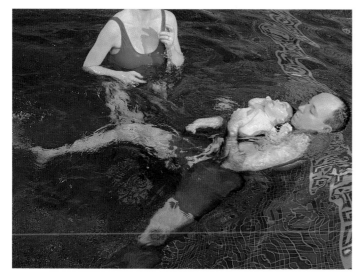

△ When you are ready to launch off, make a point of not holding your baby in a tense or anxious way.

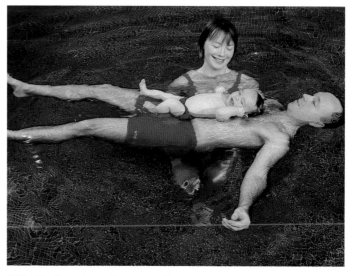

△ Floating becomes easier as you relax more. Small movements of your arms and legs ... and you are off.

From front rides to swimming

Free front rides encapsulate the spirit of enabling your baby to swim, through shared pleasure in the water and progressive independence from the support of your body. Front rides are particularly enjoyable because you can communicate all the time and guide your baby, with both eye contact and words, throughout the process of detaching herself from you. Swimming with your baby is a far more effective way of encouraging independent swimming than just holding your baby and walking in the water. The difference between the two is immediately perceived and registered by babies. Once you start swimming, there is no going back to walking.

hand floating or surfing a young baby

With a young baby who does not hold on yet, but floats on your body while you swim, you can be more daring and just support your baby's head with one hand for floating or support her chest with one hand for body surfing. This is easier than it looks, and any confident swimmer who is able to relax

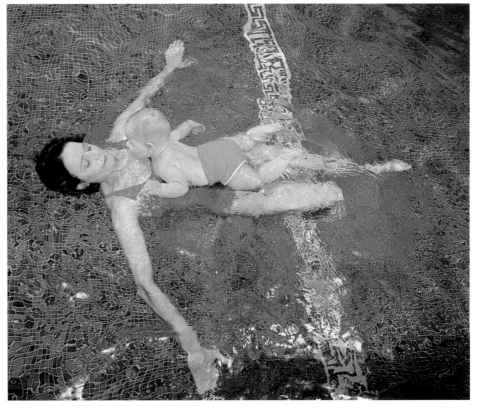

△ Once your baby has found her balance on your body, you can swim her up and down the pool.

▽ Free front rides provide opportunities for communication between parents and babies, stimulated by movement and closeness in the water.

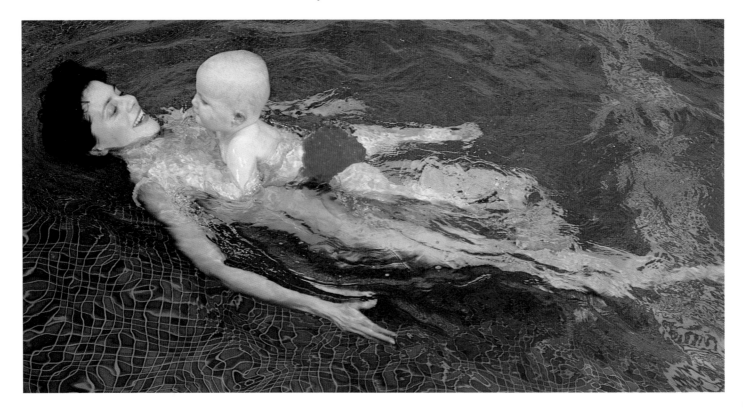

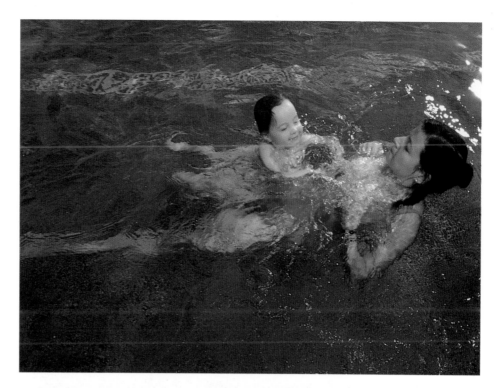

▷ Let older babies hold on only loosely to you, alternating times of rest, when they sit freely on you, with towing them along with two hands, then one hand, then one finger.

with a young baby can achieve it in one session. Babies register the difference between your standing in the pool and your swimming, and they often produce their best amphibian movements when you swim with them in this way. With practice, you become able to move your arm and bring your baby on to your body, either on her back or on her front, so that you can alternate front rides with hand floating or surfing in a relaxed way.

front towing

As you swim more and more freely with your baby in front rides, you no longer need to lift her up immediately when she slips down your body. If she is unconcerned, let her find a looser balance in which she is holding on to you less with just her head above the water. To make this even more dynamic, you can hold the hands of an older baby and let her go down further so that she is only slightly supported by your thighs. Encourage kicking as much as possible by praising her when she does it. After some time, your baby is no longer riding but

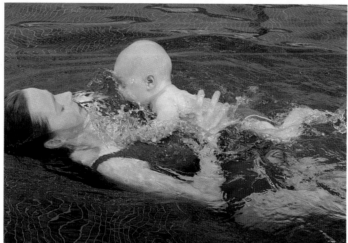

◁ Gradually let your more confident baby slide down your body for more freedom to kick.

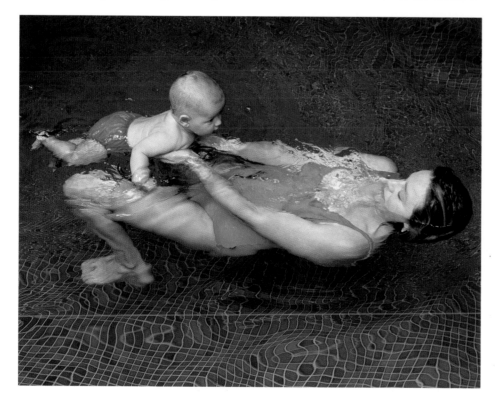

being towed in a way that invites her to make as much leg movement as possible to reach you. Make sure that this does not become frustrating, and pull your baby regularly towards you for a hearty hug. Some babies dunk their heads under the surface as they get towed and need lifting up at short intervals. One day, you may find that you can let go briefly and it has happened – she is swimming. Make sure you keep up the momentum and alternate towing and letting go to maintain your baby's self-confidence as her arm movements become stronger. Frequently a symbolic hand or finger is needed by an older baby for weeks, or months, when swimming with you.

◁ When your baby no longer enjoys being floated on her back, because she likes to lift her head up, try surfing her along as you swim on your back.

Back rides

While front rides are ideal for swimming with a young baby and towing an older baby, back rides are the most comfortable way of swimming with a baby over five months. They require more active involvement of your baby, as he needs to learn to hold on to you in some way at first.

The early reflex that makes newborns cling to their mothers is not cultivated, as we do not carry our babies enough and therefore they have to "relearn" to hold on at a later stage. Back rides are an excellent way of helping Western babies recover this skill, which Amazonian babies develop from birth. Like front rides, they are a close, intimate, yet dynamic, way of enjoying being with your baby in water.

apprenticeship

Back rides require more patience than front rides and possibly the aid of someone else to help your child hold on to you. A few babies grasp whatever they can – straps or hair – and stay on from the start. Most babies need an apprenticeship, which can take from two to six weeks. At first it may seem easier to take back rides with mothers, because their swimsuits and hair are easier to hold on to. In fact, this does not make much difference, and babies learn just as fast to hold on to their dads' backs, even though there may be nothing to cling to. Swimming breaststroke is easier for babies than crawl because the symmetrical movements facilitate stability.

Have someone at your side who is prepared to keep your baby on your upper back by placing their hands on your shoulders. Each time your child gets destabilized, your kind helper who walks along as you swim can pick him up gently and place him back in position again. With some babies, this may occur quite a few times across a training pool. Do not get discouraged, but do not try for too long. Two lengths are enough in the first two or three sessions. In the course of this apprenticeship, allowing your baby to fall off in the water once or twice may help him to register the implications of not holding on. Make sure, however, that he does not get distressed as a result. Older babies need greater care and consideration. When your baby falls off, pick him up calmly, hug him and get going again as soon as possible. With practice, your helper will only need to watch as you take off with your baby, ready to come to the rescue if needed. While some dads feel they need to hold their baby's hands at first in the back rides, this is not necessary, and it may be counterproductive to the apprenticeship of holding on.

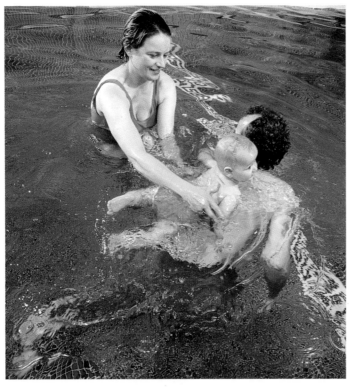

◁ **You need trust, patience and perseverance to help your baby discover that he can cling to you in comfort.**

▽ **After a variable period of apprenticeship, you no longer need your helper and can take off in mutually enjoyable rides.**

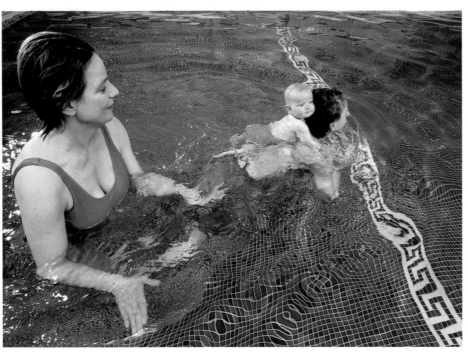

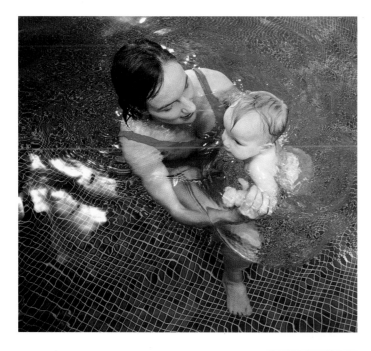

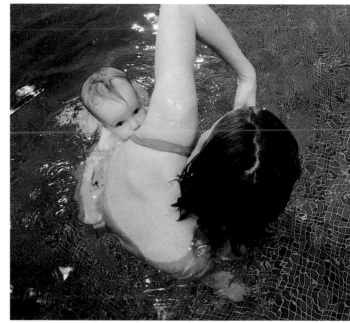

△ **Ask your baby if he is ready to go on your back for a ride, and initiate finger holding so that he can anticipate the next steps.**

positioning your baby yourself

Each parent works out a slightly different way of positioning their baby for a back ride. It may be daunting at first, but after a few trials you will be confident that you can do it. The more you are in the water, as opposed to standing up in the pool, the easier it is likely to be.

Amazonian mothers swiftly swivel their babies on to their backs, holding them from the arms. In modern pediatrics, however, this is not advisable. In the *Birthlight* classes, parents find it easier to hold their babies as for figures of eight and slide them sideways on to their backs, avoiding a lifting action. From the figures of eight, swivel your baby sideways to position him on your upper back, making sure that you take off as soon as your baby is steady. Movement helps babies to hold on and find their balance.

Allow your child to find his own most comfortable position for the stage he is at, close to your head if not very experienced, much lower down for relaxed babies.

If your baby falls off, turn around without panicking, pick him up gently, give him a hug and lift him back on again. When you wish to end the ride, get your footing in the water and reach back with your arms to bring your baby sideways in front of you for yet another hug. You can also sit your baby behind you on the edge of the pool.

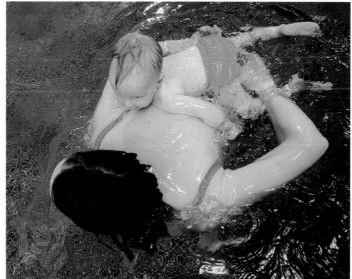

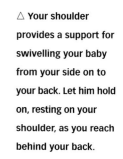

△ **Your shoulder provides a support for swivelling your baby from your side on to your back. Let him hold on, resting on your shoulder, as you reach behind your back.**

◁ **Push your baby on to your back and reach to his hands as he rests on your upper back, or let him hold on in his own way.**

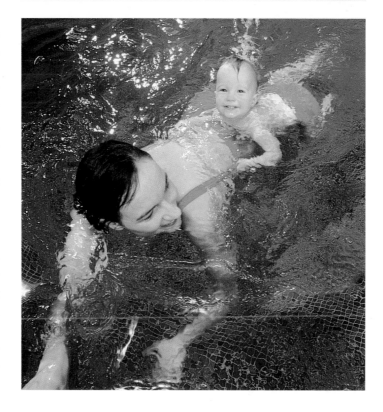

◁ **Some babies nearly strangle their parents, some ride on all fours like acrobats, others lie down in comfort. This baby enjoys swimming while he holds on to his mother.**

Enjoying back rides

After the apprenticeship stage follows a long period of enjoying back rides that extends beyond the time when your toddler can already swim unaided next to you. A desire for comfort or intimacy may prompt your baby to seek the support of your back for a while, or you may take your baby on a long crossing as a special joint adventure. Taking babies swimming does not mean that the entire focus should be on the development of their skills – there can be space for your swimming too. Even if pool regulations stop you from taking your baby into the main pool, swimming around the training pool can be more energetic than it appears and can help you return home energized. Although breaststroke is the easiest and most comfortable way to give your baby a back ride, confident babies will hold on if you prefer switching to freestyle at a later stage.

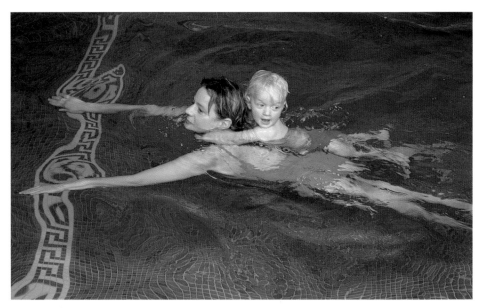

△ Toddlers find their favourite cruising style and observe what's going on in the pool as you swim.

▽ Some babies get so relaxed that they enjoy playing games, taking their hands off and clowning around on their parents' backs as they swim.

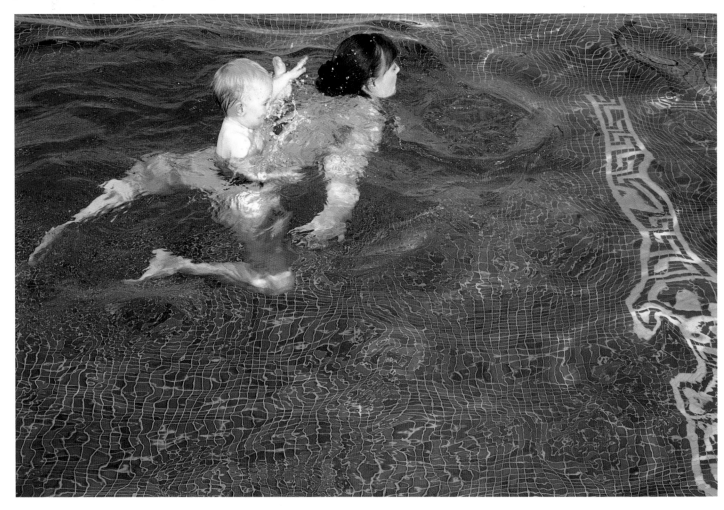

Making the most of it

Here are a few points that may contribute to your enjoyment of back rides with your baby:

- Allow your baby to find her particular favourite position on your back. Each baby will prefer to be in a position that seems to be set after some weeks of practice. Some babies are very high up, close to their parents' heads, while others are very low on the parents' backs. Some babies ride nearly upright, raising themselves on their knees in almost an all-fours position; some babies extend their arms around their parents' necks for security. There can be some changes but overall, respect the position that your baby adopts, as it is likely to be the one that suits her own needs best.

- Try and lenghten your stroke, making your movements as smooth and efficient as possible as you swim with your baby on your back. She will be registering the way you swim. Babies show a marked preference for dynamic yet regular movements, irrespective of your competence as a swimmer.

- At the same time as you swim with your baby, be aware of the harmony that develops between your two bodies in the water. Relax while you swim, making it a soothing experience for both of you. Back rides can be very calming for your baby and a quick way to renew closeness with each other – for example, after a few demanding trials of unaided swimming.

- Be responsive to your baby's feelings and moods. Is she a little sleepy right now? Then it is time for a cruise around the pool. Does she need calming down after high throws? A few steady, calm strokes may help. Is she in a playful, cuddly mode? Try a lively, more energetic stroke that will make demands on her sense of balance and delight her.

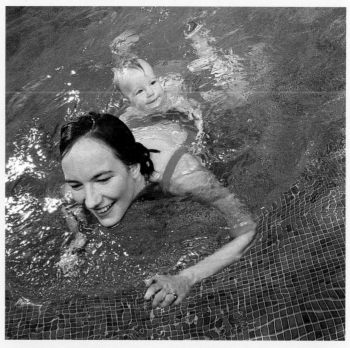

△ **Let your baby find out where and how to hold on to you. With fathers, there may not be much to hold on to, but that is fine too.**

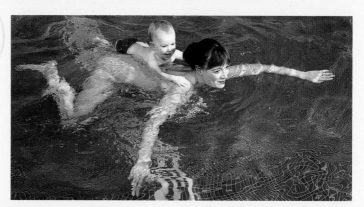

△ **Some babies like trying different positions. They may fall off, but just turn around and pick them up calmly.**

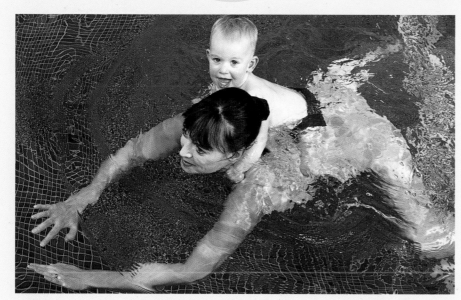

△ **When your baby is in a playful, communicative mode, she may come up and cuddle you, sometimes for a cheek to cheek swim that confirms you are her beloved parent.**

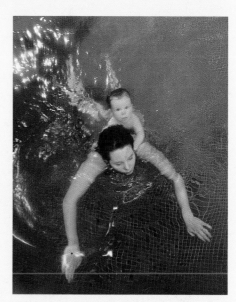

△ **Swimming with your baby can also be good swimming for you, an ideal postnatal exercise.**

Seal rides

You may have already tried front rides when you dived holding your baby in front of you. "Seal rides" are more advanced, as they require your baby to hold on steadily to you as you swim before you try and dive with him on your back. But that is all your baby needs to do. You may be surprised that your baby actually stays on your back when you take your first dive after watching other people take their babies for spectacular seal rides. As with front rides, seal rides are usually more dramatic for parents than for babies, who usually adapt easily to the underwater world. They allow parents greater freedom of movement than do front rides, since both arms and legs can be used to swim. They bond parents and babies in

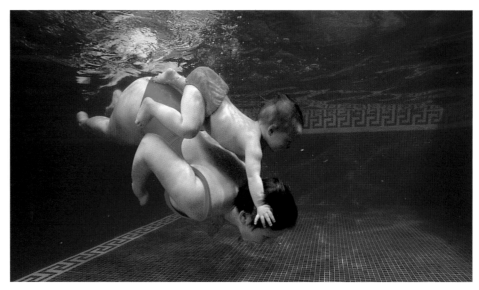

△ After your baby swims confidently on your back, he may enjoy developing diving skills, which contribute to his overall development.

Seal diving

Many babies enjoy the sense of adventure that they get from this joint activity with you. With practice, you can start taking two seal dives in succession, swimming a few strokes in between.

1 Unlike front dives, start your dive while you are swimming. With your baby on your back, signal that you are preparing to dive, and give your usual breathing signal for closure. Then boldly direct your head downwards and begin swimming underwater without stopping. In a training pool, you are likely to swim along the pool floor.

2 Surface after a couple of strokes, and gradually lengthen your dives as your baby gets used to them. Make sure that you continue swimming after surfacing unless your baby is unhappy, in which case stand up in order to hug and comfort him. Movement is key to the success of any seal dive, as it makes it easier for your baby to stay on board.

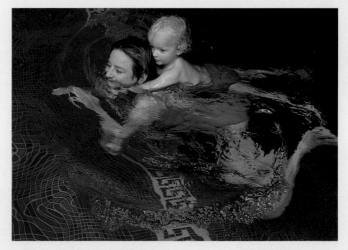

△ Before taking a seal ride, gather momentum in a few energetic strokes, making sure that your baby is steady on your back.

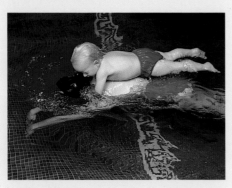

△ Lower your head and arms for a deep dive. If this is difficult, push from the floor with your feet.

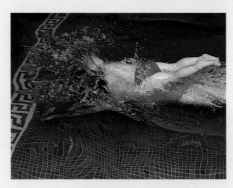

△ It takes more depth than most parents first realize to dive with your baby on your back.

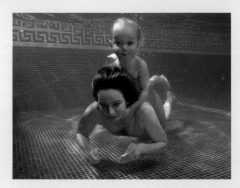

△ Surface gradually while swimming, rather than at a steep angle, which may destabilize your baby.

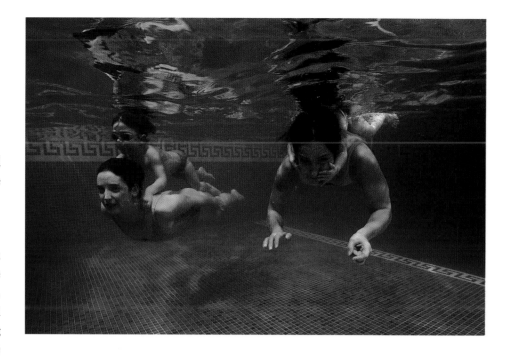

adventures that transform a training pool into another universe and perhaps leave children with long-lasting memories.

seal dive and retrieving

Once you are confident with seal dives, you and your baby can use them to retrieve objects from the bottom of the pool. During these dives, your baby picks up all the necessary information for future diving alone: estimating depth; the distance of the object; the angles of approach to it. The excitement of retrieving, while holding on to one parent through this intense movement, enables older babies and toddlers to be increasingly at ease underwater and to hold their breaths for longer. If you practised games with hoops when you started doing duckling dives, you can now reintroduce them at the bottom of the training pool.

In the *Birthlight* approach, seal dives have proved to be a sound introduction to retrieving and exploring underwater in a way that is linked to swimming. It is easier for a toddler to become used to the forward movement of a dive on a parent's back than to submerge alone, particularly if the toddler has become very buoyant. Toddlers move easily from retrieving with you in seal dives to diving by themselves. Most of them continue to enjoy seal dives until they are older. Taking them to explore shallow waters in safe areas along the seashore where the water is warm enough may prepare them for a lifelong enjoyment of diving.

POINTS TO WATCH

- It may take a few trials to find the right depth. Most parents' first dives are too shallow, and babies stay above the surface while parents think they are underwater. Babies think this is funny.
- While trying to go deep enough, you can take a dive that is too sharp and topples your baby over your head. You will realize immediately what has happened. Without panicking, pick up your child and surface. Comfort your baby if necessary.
- If you feel that you are losing your baby while you are swimming energetically along the bottom of the pool, you can extend an arm around his body to surface with him. You can also use an arm to place him back in position on your back; if he is used to swimming on your back, he will hold on to you again to complete the dive.

▽ With an experienced toddler, swimming along the bottom of the pool towards particular targets can be a great game.

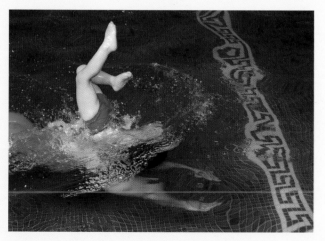

△ If you lose your baby on the dive, turn around and lift him up calmly.

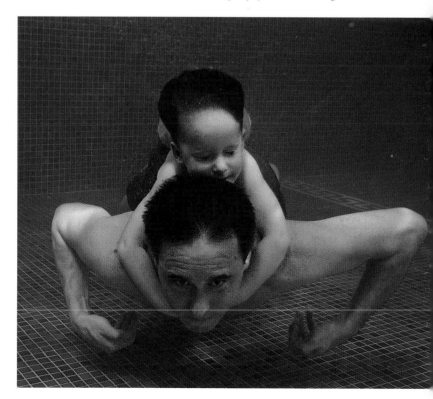

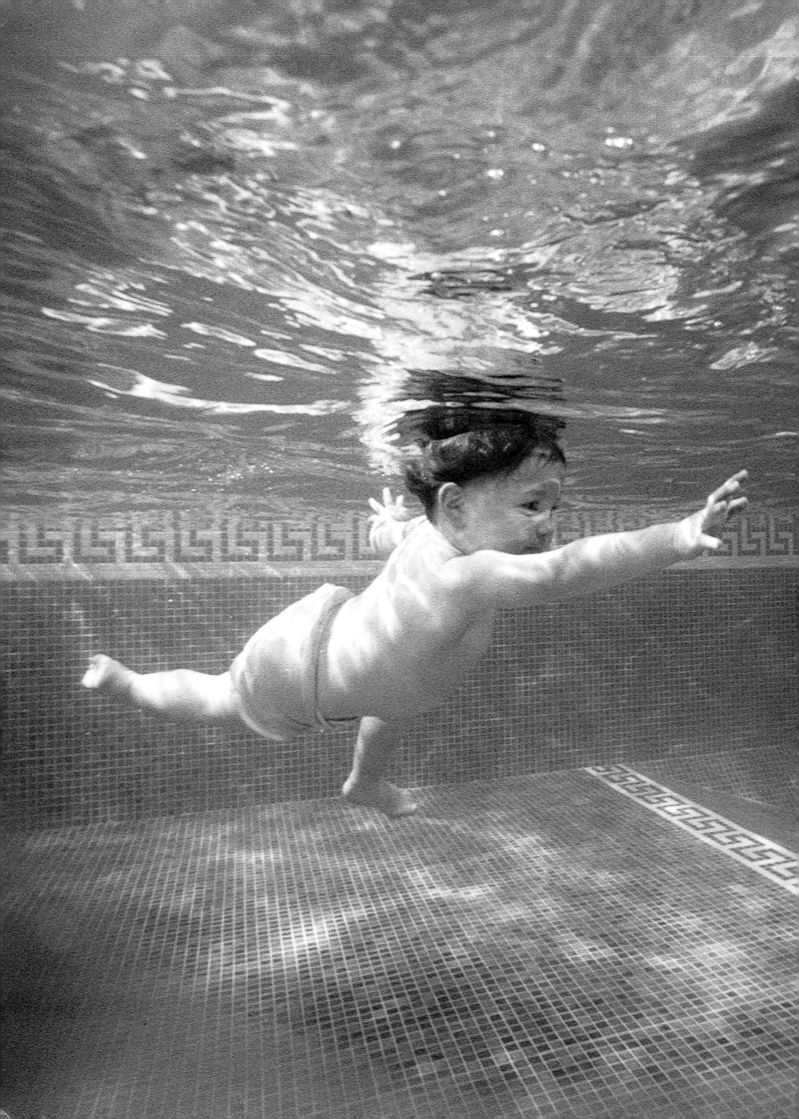

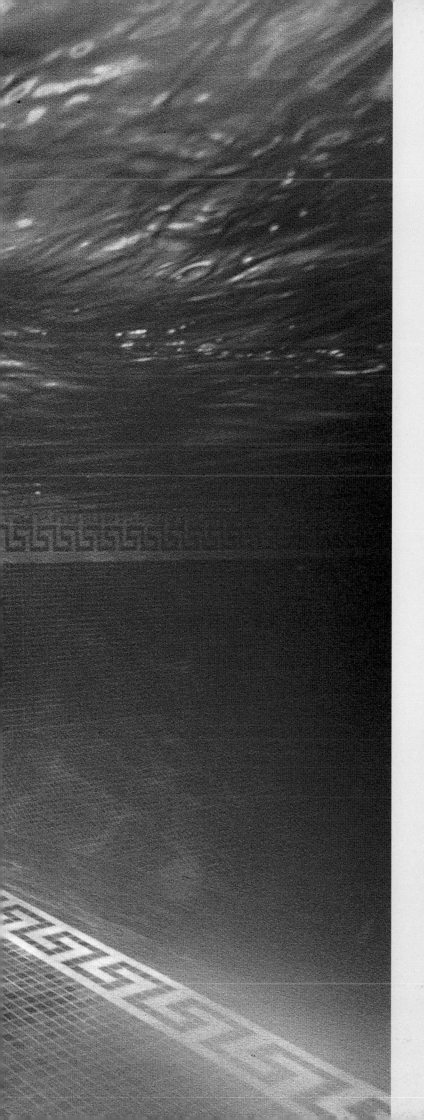

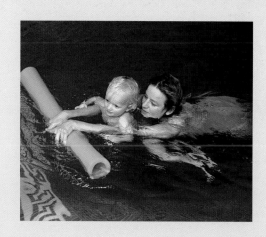

towards
swimming

Soon you will see your baby make a clear move towards swimming. You will notice that your child has become more confident and wants more independence in the water. The following exercises have been devised to help develop this confidence and independence. This is a gradual process, and every child will progress at their own pace. Eventually your child will become a fully competent swimmer, having learnt vital safety skills and a respect for the water.

Developing swimming

Swimming in a horizontal position does not come naturally to babies, who have a tendency to start propelling themselves in a vertical position in the water, with their heads just below the surface. The more strength is gained, the easier it is for babies to surface for breathing and gradually align their heads and bodies in a more horizontal position. The more relaxed babies are, the easier the pulling movement of the arms will be when they learn strokes later on. This will also result in a better body alignment.

Even if your child was "swimming" as a baby, propelling herself underwater or on her back, it is rare that a toddler is strong and co-ordinated enough to surface regularly for breathing when swimming on her front. Several techniques for strengthening and developing swimming are presented in this section. They may also help you if you began swimming with your baby late in her first year or if you have gone through all the steps but your toddler is reluctant to swim alone.

be patient

At this stage, the most important aspect of water parenting is to be detached from the goal of "teaching your baby to swim".

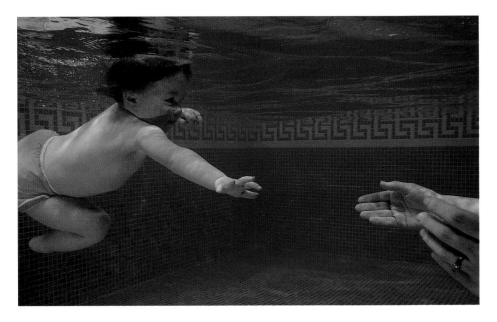

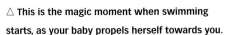

Putting pressure on your toddler to attain this goal would undermine the playful, relaxed closeness you developed earlier in the water with your baby. It may also be counterproductive to achievement. Always remember that for swimming, security and confidence are the foundations of performance and that the water environment will bring out your baby's needs and emotions. Patience and trust are perhaps the most important qualities

△ **This is the magic moment when swimming starts, as your baby propels herself towards you.**

parents can develop while their toddlers appear to be stuck forever as other babies are already swimming. Resist comparison, be steady with your weekly practice and show unconditional love. Perhaps what your toddler needs most is for you to relax and find a new game to play in the water. Then, when you no longer expect it, your toddler will decide that the time has come to show you that she can swim.

Keep safety skills in mind as your toddler develops her swimming ability. Back floating and swimming back to the edge after jumping are important skills, which you can continue practising each week. Toddlers may also take time to find their footing in shallow water. If your pool has steps, sitting on one of the top ones and having someone send your toddler to you from about 1m/3ft away can be an invaluable safety skill, given that most drowning accidents among toddlers occur in shallow water where they would have been able to stand if they had been confident enough to do so.

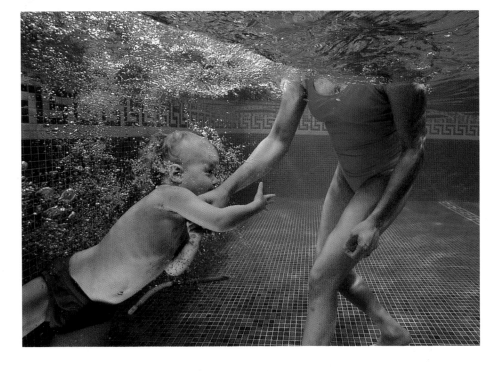

◁ **If your child is not ready to let go of you, or regresses for any reason, be patient and loving.**

Swimming to someone or something

These are the most common ways in which babies carry out the transition from swimming reflexes, when you launch your baby for a duckling dive, and conscious swimming, when she dog paddles towards you by herself.

1 Draw your baby towards you in front holding position and let her swim freely for a few seconds at a time, lifting her into your arms with a hug and praise each time.

2 Increase the distance in duckling dives, as long as your baby enjoys them. Do not repeat it if your baby finds this stressful. Many older babies and toddlers do not like swimming to anyone except their parents or siblings, or very familiar people. When your baby can propel herself for 2m/6½ft unaided, she is unlikely to be set back in her progression to fully co-ordinated swimming.

3 Toddlers may also leave the bar and swim towards you in the water. Once your baby has mastered the skill of moving along the bar, if she is happy going underwater, you can start sending her to the bar from up to 1m/3ft away, gradually increasing the distance as she develops strength as a toddler.

4 Make sure that you lavish praise for any of these breakthroughs. You have prepared for this magic moment early on, from the safety position and its variations, but do not force its occurrence. The moment will just happen suddenly one day.

5 For a long time your baby will continue to pull with bent arms and kick with bent legs, which limits the effectiveness of her movements in swimming. There is a breakthrough when toddlers start extending their arms and legs, which in the *Birthlight* approach usually occurs underwater first. Remind your baby to move her legs up and down voluntarily by using the words "kick, kick". This reminds her to make stronger and more deliberate leg movements. Now and again, move your baby's legs with your hands, and show her how you do a leg kick with plenty of splashing, which she will try and imitate.

6 Use balls or other toys to stimulate simultaneous arm pull for the strengthening of your baby's paddling action, which will continue to strengthen continuously until the third year. The development of swimming is made up of many small, mostly invisible steps which gradually give a toddler not only the physical strength and co-ordination required but also the self-confidence to take off in the water. Think of yourself as your baby's assistant, respecting her anxiety as much as celebrating her achievements.

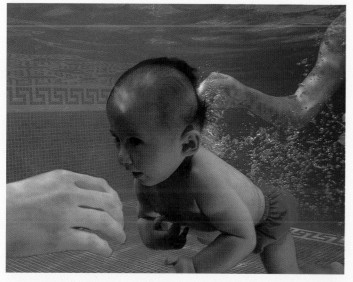

△ **Watch the transition from passive to more active dives.**

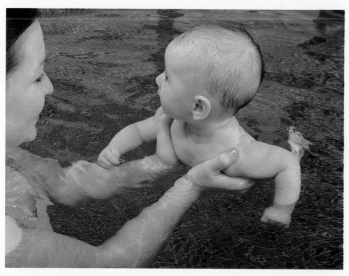

△ **One day, your baby uses her leg and arm movements to reach a target.**

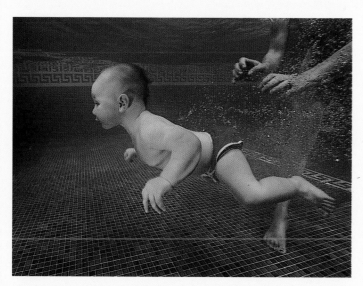

△ **Some babies develop their swimming entirely underwater.**

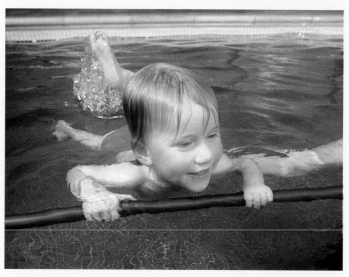

△ **Toddlers who like kicking at the bar may also enjoy a board or woggle.**

From "tugging" to swimming

At around their first birthday, some babies are reluctant to separate from their parent's body in the water; they may cling more than when they were younger. If your child enters one of these clinging phases, refusing to part from you in the water, do not attempt a forceful release. Better results are achieved by maintaining close physical contact with babies who express a strong need for it while gradually encouraging them to swim with less and less support.

close to you

Babies or toddlers who enter one of these attachment phases may refuse woggles (swim noodles) and floats, and demand to be in your arms, or at least in close contact with you rather than with anyone else, when in the water. They may show distress whenever you attempt anything different.

▽ **"Tugging" on your back allows your baby to kick freely while holding on to you for security.**

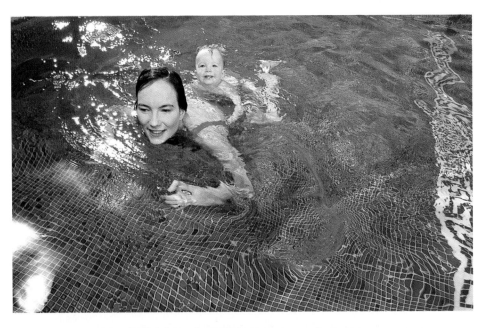

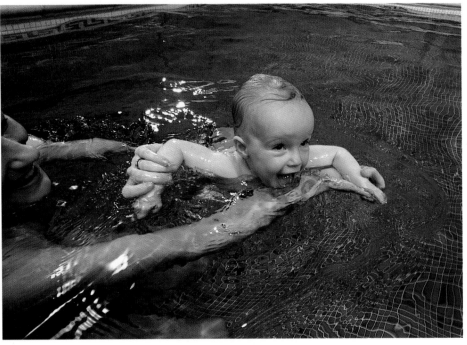

Many parents who are exposed to what appears to be a complete regression wonder whether their children have ceased to enjoy swimming – this is a time when the drop-out rate is high after promising babies look like they give up or cling, no longer their usual happy selves in the water. More than ever, this is a time to persevere and encourage your baby, week by week, even though this may be frustrating at first. The more you can relax and play, the more successfully this phase will maintain continuity with earlier highs of baby swimming. Not giving up is the challenge.

Apart from the many games you can still play – whether they include jumping and throws or not – "tugging" in various forms is probably the best way to continue developing your baby's swimming through a long clinging phase.

Tugging lets you move from swimming with your baby on your body to just holding his hand as he swims next to you. Babies who need the security of contact with you may be happy with holding a finger, a psychological more than physical support, until they are ready to take off.

When toddlers are stuck on a plateau or appear to regress, it is important to continue swimming with them regularly, encourage them through games, jumps and tugging. Should you decide to postpone swimming for a while, the benefits of your baby's early training will appear clearly later on.

tugging in breaststroke or backstroke

Let your baby drop down your back or your abdomen as low as possible to hold on comfortably. Keep good contact with your baby all the time, talking to him and, in backstroke, maintaining eye contact as well. If your baby shows anxiety, allow him to cling to you for a moment, then tug him and

◁ **Babies who refuse woggles may be happy using your arms in the same way.**

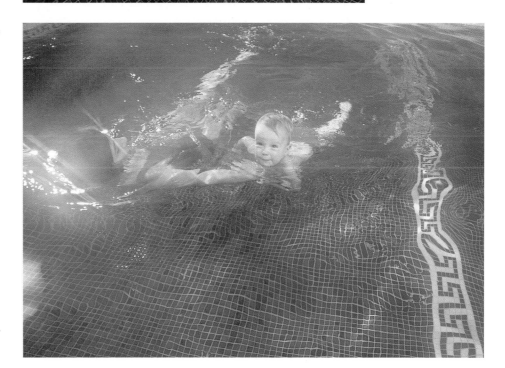

◁ While swimming
on your back, you
can tug your baby
nearly free, removing
your hands in turn
as he swims above
your body.

83

towards swimming

playfully place him back on your back or abdomen. Keep going while reassuring him that all is well and he is doing fine.

tugging with arm support

This is demanding for parents, and you may wish to use support for yourself unless you are a strong swimmer.

From the open safety position, take off on your back with your baby holding on to your open arm. You may also have your baby rest on the back of your arm and take off on your front, swimming with your legs and your other arm.

Parents can also "tug" their baby between them, holding his hands on each side while swimming across the pool.

backstroke tugging

If your baby is happy to be quite low on your abdomen, now and again – always playfully – you can try and remove one hand, then the other, at short intervals. Your baby is then effectively swimming unaided for short spells, while having the security of your body underneath his.

△ Tugging in
backstroke is not so
hard as it seems if
your baby is active,
but most parents may
need some support.

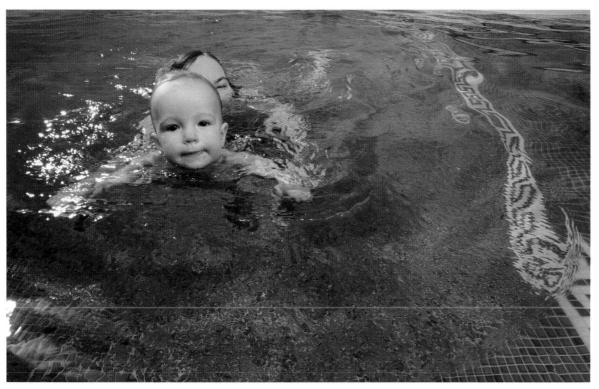

◁ When your baby is
clinging, involving him
actively in the pool
week by week – here
with a front ride – is
most conducive to
helping him in his own
unique transition
to swimming.

Swimming aids

Although very helpful as an additional source of support, swimming aids can be detrimental if babies are allowed to become dependent on them. Sometimes it is as difficult to convince a toddler to use them in order to separate from a parent as to do without them later on. Swimming aids are not absolutely necessary, and some babies and toddlers do well without them, but they help toddlers to gain strength while keeping their faces above water, and they may facilitate the transition from swimming with a parent to independence in the water.

independence in the water

Woggles (swim noodles) are versatile – lively kickers and splashers can take off in a mini-butterfly style, while cautious babies can enjoy the security of helping hands on their woggle.

Woggles help babies to develop a strong kick, and a good body alignment. They do not prevent arm movements as armbands (arm floats) do, and splashing is the best preparation for the pulling movement that babies need to develop for swimming.

woggle holding

At first, it is best to place the woggle under your baby's arms in the safety position; glide the woggle along her chest in replacement

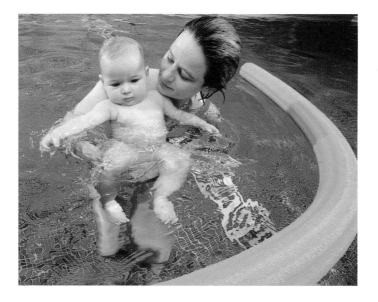

of your arm. Then place your hands on each side of your baby's arms and, if needed, help adjust her centre of gravity by making sure the woggle is tucked in under her arms rather than lower down. Start swimming as soon as possible, since movement will help your baby to consolidate her balance, with your hands on the sides of her arms, and if needed, holding her arms with your hands.

Inevitably in the first couple of weeks your baby is likely to get destabilized at some point and fall off. Pick her up gently and place her back on again in the same position, unless she is upset and needs

▷ **When you introduce woggles to your baby, whatever her age, be positive and cheerful.**

comforting. Most babies surprise their parents by getting their balance on woggles after only a few trials. When your baby is stable on her own, you may at first swim alongside her holding one end of her woggle. You can also swim on your back opposite her, encouraging her verbally to "kick" towards you, or if she is little, drag the woggle with one hand between her arms as you swim. Your baby will soon show you her favourite way of using the woggle.

Older babies are happy to hold on to a woggle and propel themselves with leg movements. As these "kicks" become

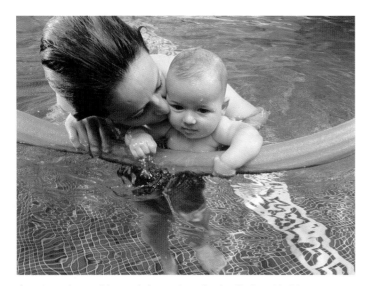

△ **Communicate with your baby as she gains familiarity with this new toy and meets a new challenge.**

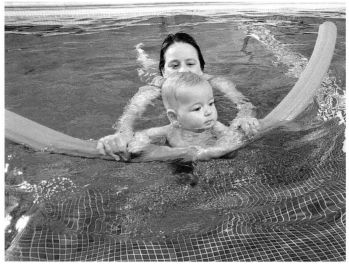

△ **Helped by movement, your baby will soon discover how to be stable on the woggle and enjoy cruising ahead.**

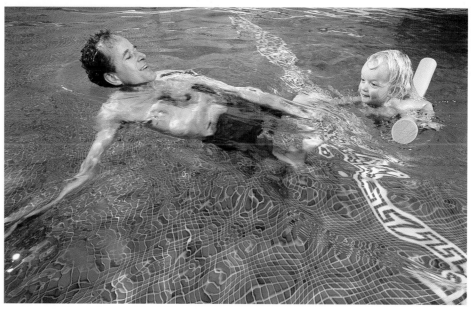

◁ With practice, your hands will no longer be needed and your baby will be stable by herself.

stronger, evolving from a reflex into deliberate movements towards a target in the pool, removing the woggle becomes a matter of time.

from little harbour to catamaran

Instead of placing a single woggle across under your baby's arms, you can also develop the little harbour into a catamaran with two woggles placed parallel under your baby's arms. At first, or if your baby needs the security of holding you, take off in the little harbour position with a woggle helping you stretch your arms in the water. Most babies over six months enjoy this ride. Two woggles – short ones are more comfortable – can then substitute your arms under your baby's arms. Catamarans are a secure transition from dependence to autonomy in the water. They are not, however, conducive to arm movements.

▽ "Tugging" with one woggle is a secure transition to swimming.

▽ This catamaran front holding with a woggle develops the little harbour in a close, secure way.

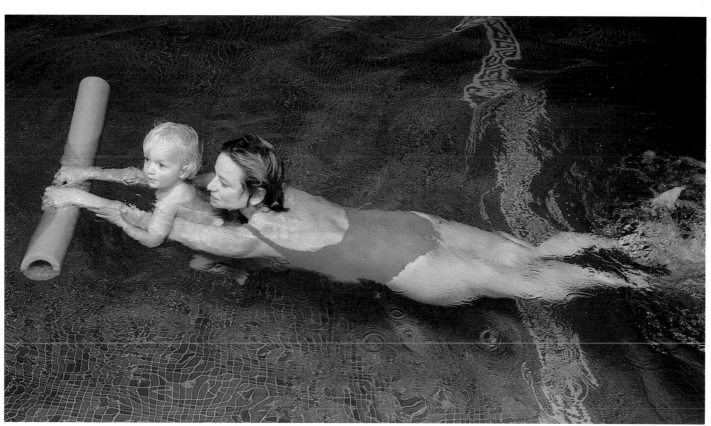

Gaining strength

When babies' arms become strong enough to pull themselves up to stand (8–14 months), their swimming enters the strengthening phase, which will enable them to cover more distance in the pool and gradually co-ordinate their arm and leg movements. Unlike the reflexive swimming movements that your baby made in the first three months, this co-ordinated action of all four limbs is now voluntary. It will take some more time, sometimes up to a whole year, for this co-ordination process to be completed to the point where your toddler will have developed his earlier dog paddle into an idiosyncratic stroke efficient enough to take him across a teaching pool.

strengthening can be practised

• In dives, use a target such as a toy, your face or your open arms underwater. Give your baby a nudge to help reach the target or a finger to pull on. Do not do it too soon, however, to allow your baby the excitement of personal self-reliant triumph.

• In swimming to the pool wall to hold on to the edge or the grab bar, on the first

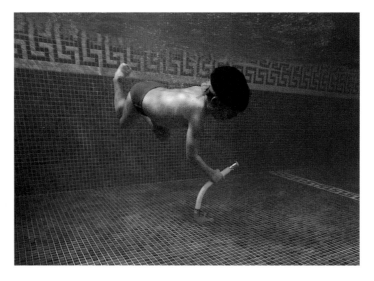

◁ Underwater swimmers who are not yet able to surface to breathe gain strength by swimming to reach toys.

attempts, the baby may come back to you after reaching the wall. Try again, and praise your baby when he gets hold of the edge or the bar, as this may be the beginning of learning how to surface to breathe. Place a toy for him to reach. If your baby keeps trying to swim back towards you after reaching the wall instead of grabbing hold of the edge or bar, follow him and gently lift him up to hold the edge or the bar, placing his hands on it and then praising him.

• Preliminary stroke instruction can begin from three years for children who have been prepared following the sequences presented in this book. Small children who have been introduced to the water early are stronger imitators of swimming drills and follow instructions in the water more easily than newcomers.

▽ Swimming to the pool edge is made easier by having something in sight near the bar or gully.

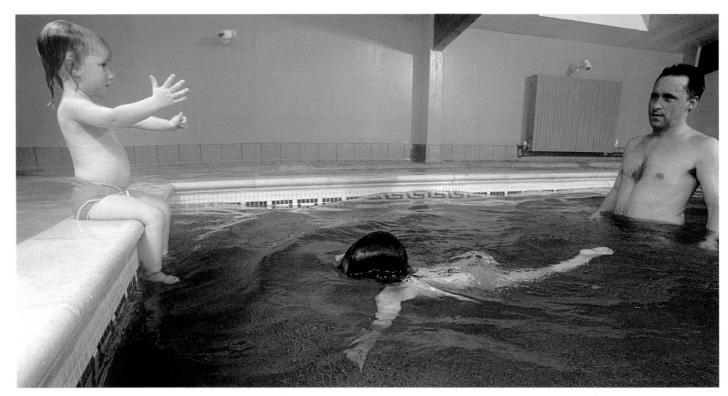

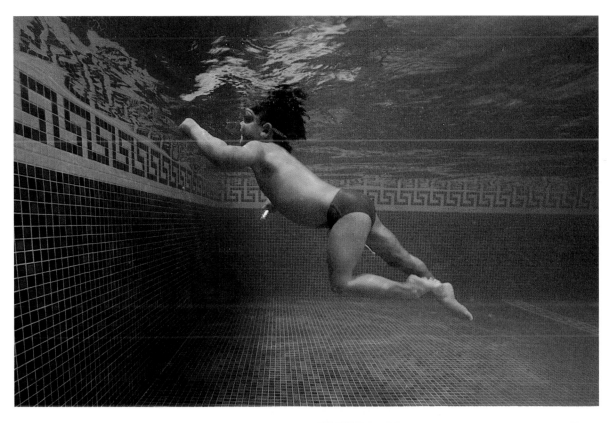

△ Early swimming requires a strong "pulling" action of the arms as well as vigorous kicking in order to surface at the pool's edge.

A lot of communication between parent and child in the water means that it is possible for a parent to alternate between teacher and playmate without contradiction. Water offers the perfect environment to swap these roles again and again within minutes, to the great delight of your child.

Strengthening requires coaxing, patience, renewed stimulation, creating excitement, but mainly promoting self-motivation to expand skills. This means introducing more games, swimming with friends and, most of all, enjoying your small child's personality as it evolves in the water. Chase games are popular with toddlers, and both boys and girls like to play shark, seal, dolphin, or a marine version of any animal they fancy. Taking your child to the zoo or water park to watch aquatic mammals at play can be very inspiring. Two year olds also register images from animal videos, and will try and imitate them in the pool.

At this stage, toddlers can also be inspired and motivated by older children. Enrol little swimmers for a water party that your toddler will be keen to be part of. Many children like swimming with babies, and are gentle and patient with them. Grandparents offer another source of stimulation. In *Birthlight* classes, the "family and friends" sessions make babies feel that swimming is part of life.

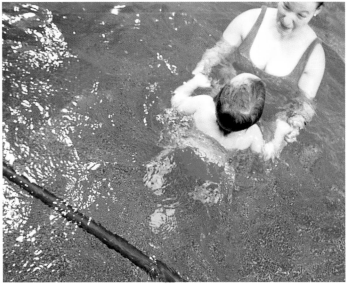

◁ Your baby will love the feeling of movement as you tow him gently through the water, allowing him to practise leg kicks.

▽ Encouraging children to play with their favourite inflatable water animals enhances their confidence and builds their strength.

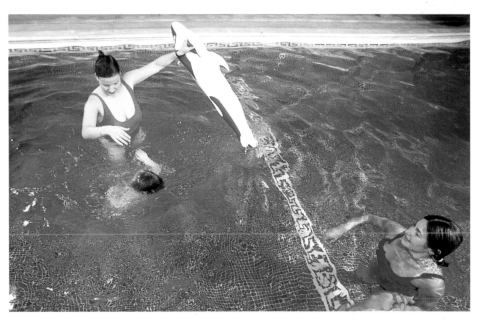

Surfacing and rolling to breathe

Surfacing to breathe happens spontaneously by strengthening the leg kick and pulling the arms as your toddler develops both greater muscular strength and increased co-ordination of the leg and arm movements. Although it is currently held that children under six are rarely able to control their breathing when they swim, small children who have started swimming as babies and continue developing their swimming into strokes, learn rhythmical breathing spontaneously as they swim, surfacing at intervals that best suit their swimming. There are two ways of surfacing: encouraging your baby to lift her head or to roll, or try both and see which one she finds easier. Both are taught skills. Rolling is more complex but more efficient for babies who do not mind being on their backs. Some babies will develop the two skills simultaneously and use them indifferently.

head lifting

If your baby is under 18 months old, it is better to help her manually to lift her head as she swims underwater. Lift your baby's chin up for breathing, signal and let her go under again without losing her swimming momentum. Start once or twice at most. After a few weeks, check if your baby can now lift her head by herself. Your baby may cover 5m/16ft, sometimes more if she is a

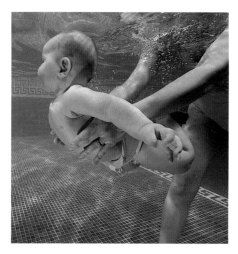

△ From the start, you train your baby to surface as you lift her up gently in front holding.

strong kicker. Have one long swim per session only, as it is a strenuous exercise. With a toddler approaching a second birthday, you can gradually aim at covering a greater distance. You can use chin lifts, if you feel they are needed, but it is better to show your baby how to kick up to the surface by your side, or to hold her under the arms and lift her just enough to surface to breathe. Whatever works will bring a huge sense of accomplishment as your baby becomes ready to cross a small pool unaided or with very little help. Make sure you celebrate this breakthrough – it may boost your baby's confidence not only at the pool but in all other aspects of development.

advantages and disadvantages of lifting the head

- It is spontaneous. Toddlers discover the way of kicking themselves up to surface and breathe.
- Some babies go vertical and then flip their heads backwards so that their face is out of the water and they can breathe. It serves the purpose but slows them down a lot.
- It is difficult for a small child to turn her head to breathe. By lifting her head she loses her alignment in the water, which should receive priority for the development of freestyle. This can be corrected to some extent by encouraging "splashing kicks" in a prone position.
- Toddlers get tired quickly from lifting their heads, and the effort causes their legs and feet to drop at first until a stronger leg movement helps to realign their bodies after lifting their heads.

rolling over to back

After your baby ceases to want to lift herself up, later in her first year, she can roll over and resume floating. This gives your baby a way of resting and breathing freely in the water with her face up, which can be an important safety skill in the transition time before unaided swimming is established and sufficient strength has been acquired. It anticipates the rolling of the head in front crawl, and will make it easier for your baby to master rhythmical surfacing when moving from dog paddle to formal crawl. Continuing the earlier rolling from safety position to back float, you can help your nearly swimming toddler to roll over so that her face surfaces to get a breath. Your baby will soon enjoy rolling over without any help and may take to what *Birthlight* children have called "dancing in the water", that is rolling from front to back and back to front again. Some toddlers enjoy this greatly

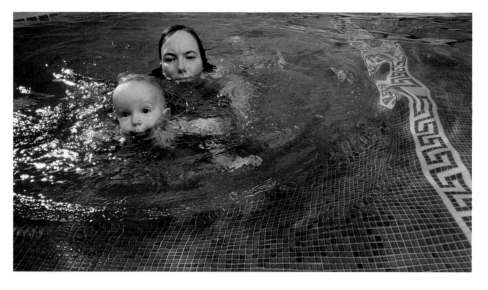

◁ While swimming with your baby or "tugging", you can tilt her sideways for rolling over.

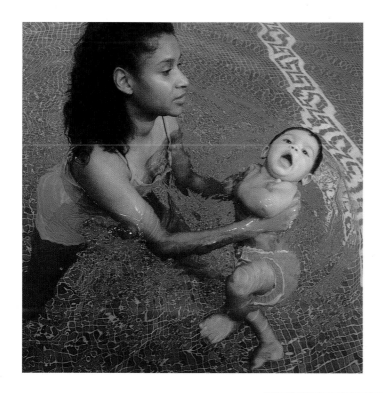

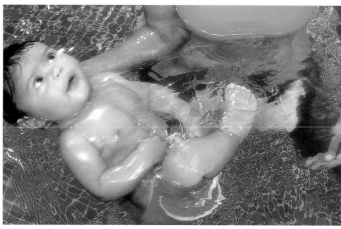

△ **In back floats, babies may enjoy playing with their feet and "talk" as they float.**

◁ **From the safety position, you can roll your baby over on to her back, roll her again on your arm, and so on and so forth as a game.**

in "water discos" with music. Do not forget to roll your baby over on her back after attempts at unaided swimming, which make her tired, for a fun rest with a supported float hold, as when she was little, or to have a hug.

While most babies tend to roll from their front on to their back unwittingly when they lose their balance in the water, doing it deliberately requires practice. Each baby has her preferred side for rolling over. Very few toddlers manage to get back again to their front until their swimming has become much stronger.

advantages of unaided rolling

- It improves babies' balance in the water, helping to preserve a horizontal position and to strengthen their arm movements.
- It makes it easier for babies to breathe freely for longer, providing a useful survival skill between early stages of unaided swimming and confident swimming.
- It is a foundation for both freestyle and backstroke.
- The main disadvantage is that rolling interrupts swimming and many toddlers find the combination challenging.

backstroke

Practising floating on the back complements your baby's development and encourages simultaneous arm and leg movements after you progressively withdraw head support.

STARFISH

Playing "starfish" is a good exercise to encourage backstroke. Using two woggles, one under each arm, let your toddler propel herself on her back. Woggles allow toddlers to stay afloat without facing the challenge of floating alone.

▷ **On two woggles, toddlers are in control. Show them how to kick and splash with their feet.**

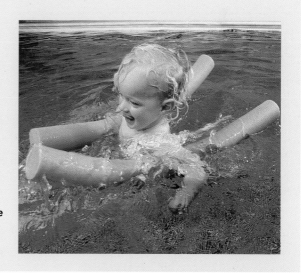

Some babies enjoy swimming on their backs early in life; others dislike it until much later. Ask your child to look at you so that she aligns her whole body on the surface of the water. Holding a board on her tummy with both her arms can also help your toddler to continue relaxing while in water.

When it is time to send your child to a swimming class in which you will not be in the water any longer, celebrate that step as the completion of a happy process. Family swimming sessions can continue, and during them, your child will enjoy showing you her latest accomplishments in the water. Having fun in the water together can be an enjoyable experience for many years to come, and you may find that you develop a shared enjoyment of many water sports.

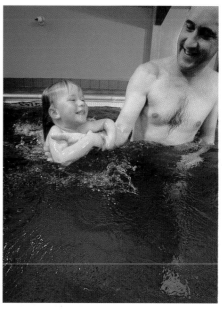

△ **Skills do not matter as much as a happy child and shared quality time.**

Diving games

Water babies grow up to be at ease in water – swimming, diving and playing both on the surface and underwater. Diving games reaffirm a positive playful attitude from the first duckling dive until you are amazed to see your small child take off to explore the underwater world by herself.

help your child take a dive

From early on, teaching your baby to dive from a sitting position on the pool side or on a float can be very good for confidence building. Your baby dives towards you, and you are there to lift her up and hug her. All diving games develop this early experience, which your baby consolidates in many ways through duckling dives, front holding dives and seal dives. If your child is nearly one or if you introduce a toddler to water, reaffirming games with diving are most important to help secure her confidence on each visit to the pool. Be very patient and respectful of your toddler's resistance while also confidently showing her the way.

From the moment a toddler can jump from a standing position, be very firm about where to dive and where not, so that she associates diving with having the "go-

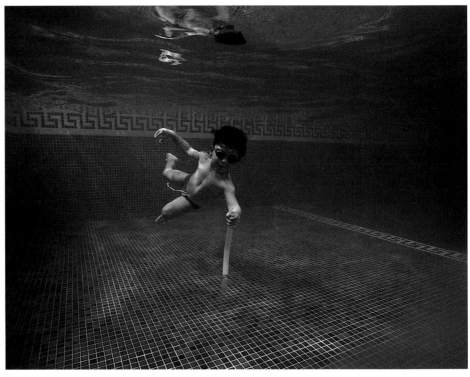

△ Solo retrieving marks your baby's accomplishment as an early swimmer in his third year. After throwing a target, he dives confidently, swims towards it and brings it proudly to his watchful parents.

ahead" from an adult. This is important for later, in case of shallow or unsuitable water.

Both babies and toddlers best learn to dive by themselves from floats. You can also help a toddler to bring her arms together

above her head while sitting on the pool side with her feet on the grab bar or in the gully, look down and go. Let your baby regulate her own diving. Some babies enjoy repeated dives, others need longer intervals. If your baby chokes, cuddle her and let her decide the right time to go under again.

diving for treasure

This is one of the games that a toddler who is happy jumping into the pool by herself enjoys the most, as it gives her a feeling of independence and special achievement.

Once your child is comfortable underwater for a few seconds at a time, mastering further breath control with a goal is a favourite game that leads to deep-water enjoyment. It can be easier for a two year old to propel herself underwater towards a goal than to dog paddle to a floating toy. In

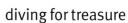
◁ The foundation for diving games is made of the consolidated trust your baby has gained with each early jump and duckling dive.

▷ After throwing your target object, take a
deep dive with your toddler, holding him with
one arm by your side.

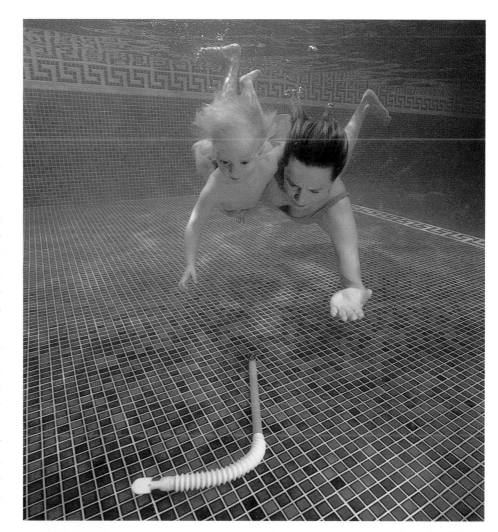

chlorinated pools, it is advisable to buy a
pair of goggles at this stage. Goggles also
give your child clearer vision underwater.

Throw an object into the water and wait
until it sinks to the bottom. Let your toddler
retrieve it and return triumphantly to the
surface. The objects must be colourful and
easy to grasp – a toy that is only just heavy
enough to sink adds to the fun since your
child can pick it up in mid-water.

Place some weighted plastic toys at the
bottom of the pool or use the colourful
rings supplied at many pools. Let your child
throw an object and watch it sink before
diving for it.

Take your child under, in a front dive or
seal dive, and put the object in her hand
before surfacing. In time, she will confidently
take the object by herself. Infants soon realize
how much this skill impresses adults.

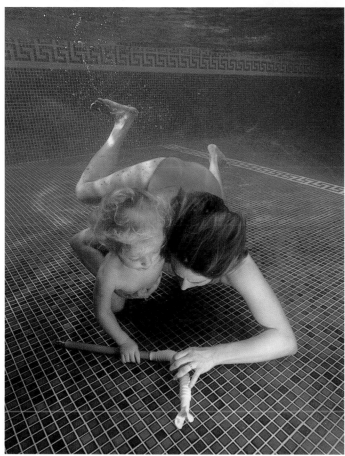

△ Your child may reach the object at the same time as you, but placing it
firmly in his hand ensures success.

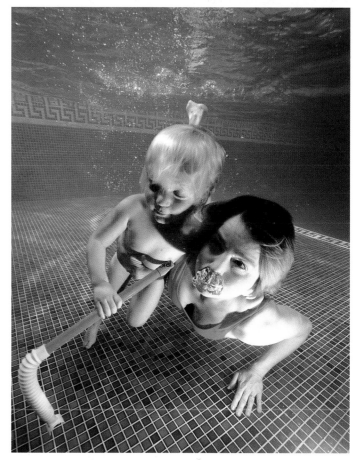

△ Breathe out gradually as you swim to the surface with your child and
the object. He will enjoy showing others how he got hold of it.

Typical session formats

This book highlights the many ways in which your baby may make the transition from early amphibian reflex movements to co-ordinated swimming. Following the process from a baby's first introduction to the pool to the first few metres/feet of unaided dog paddle is an especially rewarding experience for every parent, which more than compensates for the time and dedication required. Session formats differ for babies under six months, who are still absorbed in their experience of being in water close to you, and babies over six months, who can hold on to you and gradually enjoy developing motor skills.

Starting under six months

For a young baby, comfort and closeness are of prime importance for creative, positive associations with baby swimming. Remember that being in water with you is a rich multi-sensory experience for your baby. What you do in the pool is not so important as how you do it. While you float your baby, make sure that you can relax and be fully with her. Whether you are an avid swimmer or barely water-confident, the more relaxed you are, the freer your baby will be to move in the water. Decisive and firm, yet calm and steady movements are essential for successful submersion. Quitting on a happy note and avoiding overtiredness are desirable.

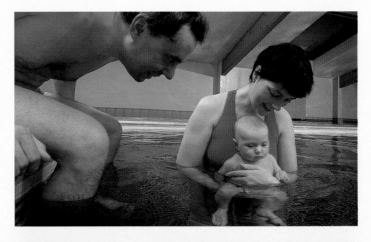

▷ **Be relaxed together and enjoy closeness in the water.**

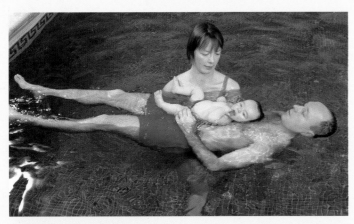

△ **Enjoy lots of love-bonding.**

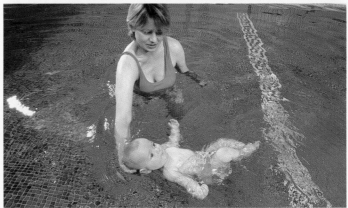

△ **Strengthen swimming reflexes in various positions, front and back.**

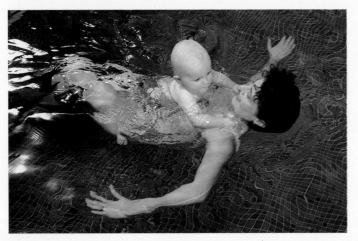

△**Swim freely with your baby on your front.**

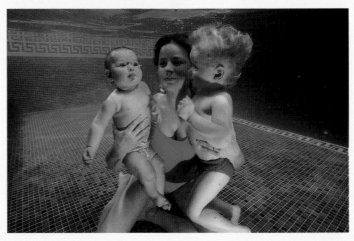

△ **Make your baby at ease with submersion.**

Starting over six months

The older babies are when you take them swimming, the more you have to tailor sessions to their budding personalities. Have you got an impulsive, carefree baby who throws herself into the water or a very cautious baby who needs convincing that, all things considered, this might be fun? Babies over six months need movement, variety and games in short succession. Use woggles and floats to swim with your baby and promote self-reliance. Sessions need to be action-packed, alternating jumps and dives with swimming. Apart from practising ways of holding, swim rather than walk whenever you can. Rituals are important to ensure continuity; pay attention to the way you begin and end sessions, and pack toddlers their favourite snacks.

▷ Build self-confidence and gradually self-reliance in the water through closeness, communication, trust, play and lots of praise.

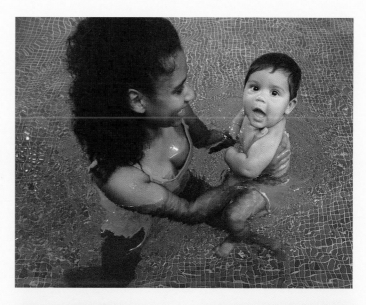

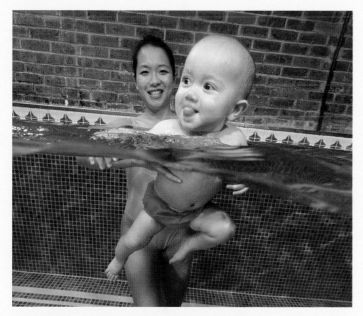

△ Encourage leg and arm movements for swimming.

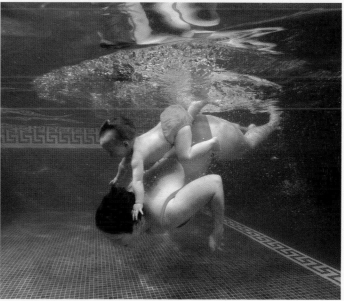

△ Increase breath-holding capacity underwater.

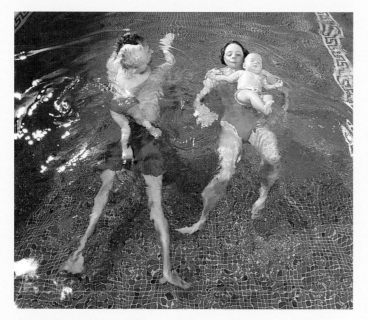

△ Swim freely with your baby on your front and back, and progressively detach your baby from your body, with or without swimming aids.

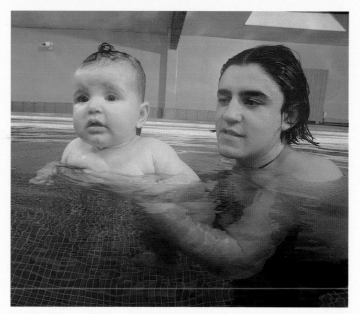

△ Develop safety skills.

Resources and acknowledgements

Useful addresses

UK ADDRESSES

Amateur Swimming Association
(the official UK swimming association)
Harold Fern House
Derby Square
Loughborough
Leicester
LE11 0AL
Tel (01509) 618700

Birthlight & Aqualight
(Postnatal Aqua Yoga, Baby Waves classes
and training programme in the UK)
7 Essex Close
Cambridge
CB4 2DW
Tel/Fax (01223) 362288
www.birthlight.com
www.aqualight.co.uk

Little Dippers Club
(Lauren Heston's infant water safety training)
South Point House
8 Paston Place
Brighton
BN2 1HA
Tel (01273) 639622

Splashdown Waterbirth Services
17 Wellington Terrace
Harrow on the Hill
Middlesex
HA1 3EP
Tel (020) 84229308

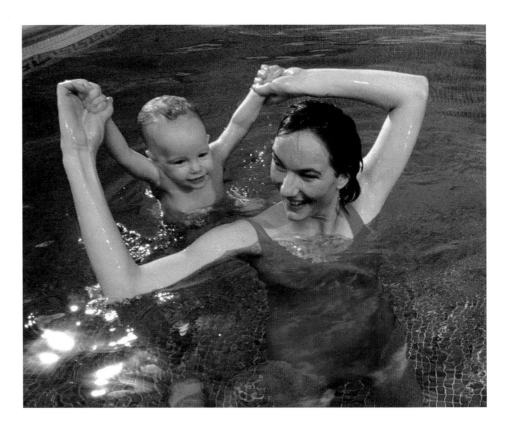

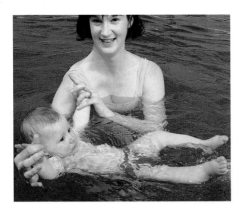

US ADDRESSES

Amateur Swimming Association
1 Olympic Plaza
Colorado Springs
Colorado, 80909
Tel (001) 719 578 4578

**American Swimming Coaches
Associations & Swim America**
2101 North Andrews Avenue, Suite 107
Fort Lauderdale, Florida 33311
Tel (001) 954 563 4930

Waterbirth International
PO Box 1400, Wilsonville
OR 97070
Tel (001) 503 682 3600
Toll free 1 (800) 641 baby
www.waterbirth.org

World Aquatic Babies Congress
5508 Britton Drive, Long Beach
California 90815
Tel (001) 310/198 0235
www.waterbabies.org

OTHER ADDRESSES

Canadian Swimming
1600 James Naismith dr., Suite 503
Gloucester, Ontario, Canada KB1B 5N4
Tel: (001) 613 748 5673

South African Federation
(Swimming South Africa)
245 Admiral's Court, Tywhitt, Mall,
Rosebank, P.O. Box 1608
Saxonworld 2132
Johannesburg, South Africa
Tel: (0027) 11 880 4328

Australia Swimming Inc.
Room 7, Act Forthouse
100 Maitland Street
Hackett, Act 2602, PO Box 940
Australia
Tel: (00612) 6257 4837

New Zealand Swimming Federation
65 Victoria Street, Level 4, Central Library
Wellington , New Zealand
Tel: (0064) 447 30 383

Further reading

Swim, Baby, Swim, Hawley, Ann
(Pelham Books, London, 1989)

Water Baby! a first fun book of water skills,
Heston, Lauren (Element Children's Books, 1999)

Teaching an Infant to Swim, Hunt, Newman, Virginia
(Angus & Robertson Publishers, 1985)

We are all Water Babies, Johnson, Jessica & Michel
Odent (Dragon's World Ltd, 1994)

References

Elsner, R. & B. Gooden, *Diving and Asphyxia* (detailed
coverage of the diving response), Monographs of the
Physiological Society No. 40, Cambridge, MA, USA:
Cambridge University Press, 1983.

Galbraith, N.S., "Infections associated with swimming
pools", *Environmental Health* 88:31-33, 1980.

Goldberg, G.N. et al, "Infantile water intoxication after
a swimming lesson", *Pediatrics* 70(4):599-600, 1982.

Johnson, P. "Birth under Water: to breathe
or not to breathe" (review article), *British Journal of
Obstetrics and Gynaecology* 103:202-208, 1996.

McGraw, M.B. "Swimming behaviour of the human
infant", *Journal of Pediatrics* 15, 485-90, 1939.

Suk Ki Hong, "Breath-hold Diving" in A.A. Bove
and J.C. Davis Eds, *Diving Medicine* W.B. Saunders
Company 1990 (second edition): 58-68.

Van Dyk, D. *Water Safety for Infants: the Drownproofing
Method* (for counter-reference only), Landsdowne
Press, Melbourne, 1975.

Wennergren, G. et al, "Laryngeal Reflex", Acta
Paediatrica, Supplement 389:53-56, 1993.

From the author

The photography shoots for this book took place in Cambridge during the winter. It took inspiration, trouble-shooting skills and good humour from everyone involved, besides gallons of tea and hot soup, to keep the babies happy in the water. First thanks go to Ruscha Schorr-Kon for her warm welcome as we invaded not only the pool but also the playroom and the house at the Wood. The memory of Stephan Schorr-Kon was held vividly. Warm thanks to Christine Hanscomb and her team for beautiful surface and underwater photographs, which convey the love exchanged between parents and babies in water. Sue Duckworth's array of skills as a stylist deserve special credit. Whenever anything or anyone needed fixing, Drake was there. It took the co-ordination and talent of both Debra Mayhew and Melanie Halton, who took over the editing when Debra went on maternity leave, to make a book from my scribbles and a heap of photographs. This book springs from years of *Birthlight* classes at the Windmill School pool; special thanks to Geoff Barnes for managing it with a heart of gold and to all the parents and babies who helped refine the approach over the years. Thanks to Sally Lomas, Louise Pivcevic, Tricia Beaumont and Amanda Walker for their support as co-teachers. My inspiration is the gratitude of a lifetime to my parents for whole summers of "messing about in the water" in the Loire, to the Amazonian families who showed me what is possible and to my four water babies, Lucia, Mary, David and Luke, who all discovered early on how to swim in different ways.

Thank you to the models

Many thanks to the families who gave up their time to help in the making of this book.

Myriam Baldor and John Norman with Matthew (2 years) and George (5 months); Gemma Barbieri with Alicia (4 months); Kate Barker with Samuel (7 months); Patricia Beaumont with Jacob (7 months); Idit and Nick Duncan with Adam (3 years) and Mia (6 months); Alison and Charlie Gilderdale with Alice (2 years) and Phoebe (4 years); Sarah Gostick with Isobel (8 months); Becky Grant with Charlie (6 months); Melanie and Simon Hamilton Davies with Manon (4 months); Liat and Evan Jones with Ariel (5 weeks); Suzy Kay with Toby (1 year); Lynne Kindell with Alice (13 months); Kate Lavender and Frank Sanchez with Daniella (5 months); Lucinda Lawrence with Samuel (4 months); Sally Lomas with Aaron (2 years); Yasmin Marsh with Jamie (5 months); Mary Jane O'Sullivan with Dominic (5 months); Jill Patterson with Emily (6 weeks); Judith and Mark Pawson with Kai (5 weeks); Judith Stanton with Becky (2 years); Hester Tingey with Bathsheba (3 weeks); Mai Ward and Rebecca Freemantle with twins Ruby and Honour (7½ months); Penny Wright with Chad (7 months).

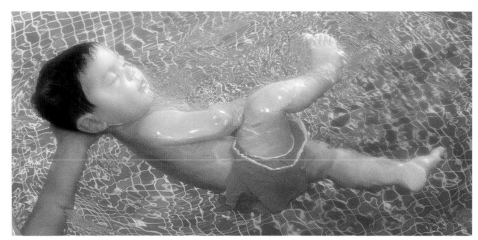

Index

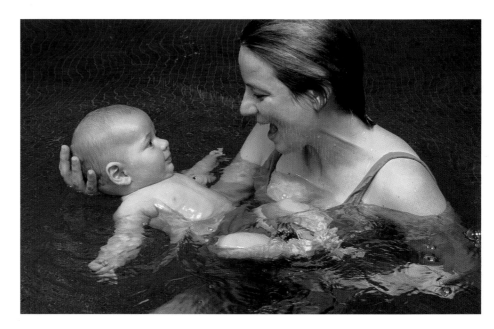

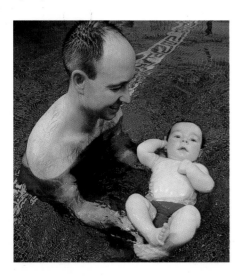